LIVE WELL

the ayurvedic way to health and inner bliss

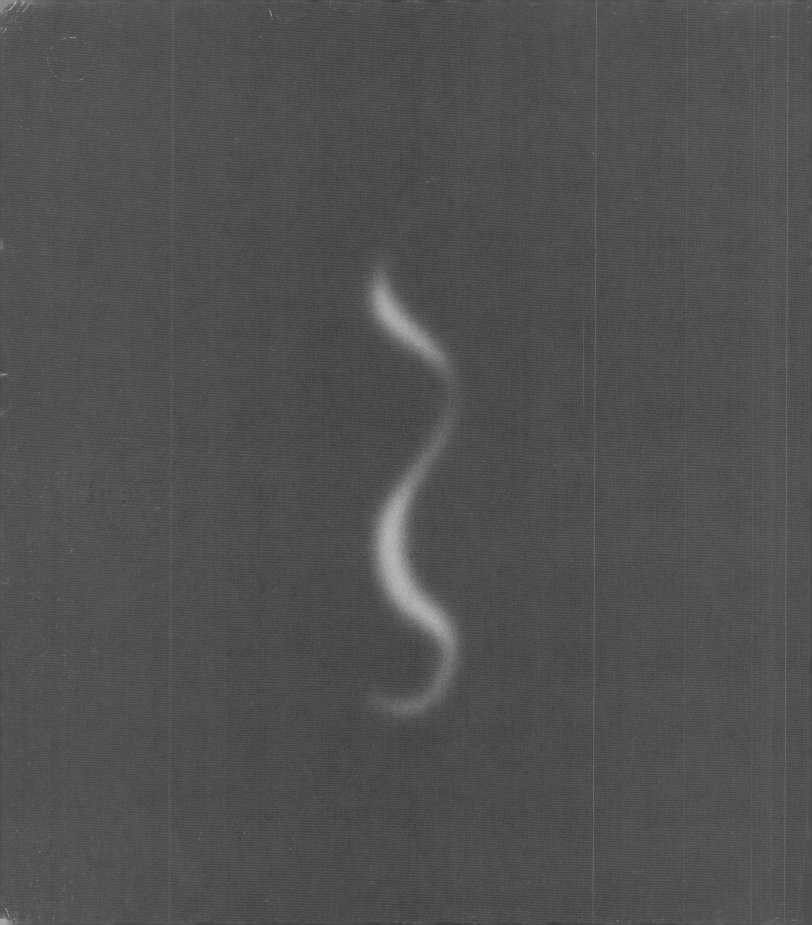

LIVE WELL
the ayurvedic way to health and inner bliss

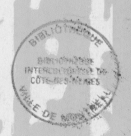

JANE ALEXANDER

ELEMENT

Element

An Imprint of HarperCollins Publishers

77–85 Fulham Palace Road

Hammersmith, London W6 8JB

10 9 8 7 6 5 4 3 2 1

Illustration on page 161 by Joan Corlass

A catalogue record for this book

is available from the British Library

ISBN 0 7225 4052 3

Printed and bound in Hong Kong

Editor: Jillian Stewart

Design: Design Revolution, Brighton.

Picture credits: Powerstock (Zefa) title page, 27, 37, 47, 86, 96, 118, 139, 145, 154;

Mary Evans xi; Digital Vision xii, 123, 136, 146; Photodisc 32; Images/Telegraph

52, 54, 150-151; Photonica 142, 165

acknowledgements

Grateful thanks go to the wonderful people who have fostered my interest in ayurveda over the last ten years and who have taught me so much. In particular, I'd like to thank Angela Hope-Murray, Dr Doja Purkit, Judith Morrison, Colin Beckley, Andrew Johnson, and Ian and Carole Hayward. And special thanks to vastu shastra practitioner Kajal Sheth.

CONTENTS

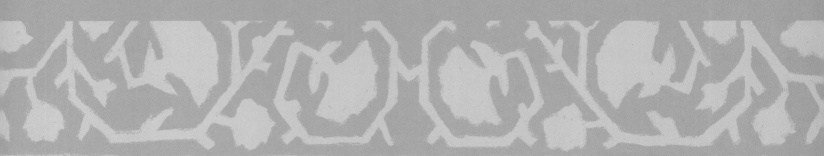

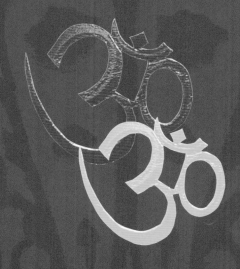

introduction

Ayurveda can change your life. There's no question about it. Follow simple rules for everyday living and you can restore yourself to nigh-on perfect health. Without undue effort you can reach your ideal weight. Within a short span of time you can be fitter, healthier, more energetic than you have ever been before. You can even fine-tune your emotions, banish stress, and find a deep sense of peace within your soul. The ancient texts even hint at that most elusive of goals – immortality or, at the very least, extreme longevity.

Ayurveda is, without doubt, the most ancient system of medicine known to humankind. It is at least 5,000 years old; some say even older. It has been called "the Mother of Medicine" and is perhaps the greatest form of healing and natural healthcare the world has ever known. Yet, until recently, ayurveda had been ignored in the West. Although it is now becoming more popular, particularly for its wonderful beauty treatments, many people are still unaware of the full powers of this extraordinary system of healthcare. Why? The answer lies in the fact that traditional ayurveda is Eastern to its very roots. Few Westerners have learned its secrets and so much of its teaching remains in Sanskrit or couched in unfamiliar and inaccessible language. Because ayurveda was suppressed for many years under hostile governments, it has not had the opportunity of being updated for the modern world. Many Westerners have been under the misconception that in order to enjoy the benefits of ayurveda you had to listen to strange Eastern music, endure unpleasant purgatory therapies, and subsist on a diet of curries. This may have been the case in the past but now all that is about to change.

This book offers all the benefits of ancient ayurveda but makes it totally accessible to modern Westerners. It explains the theory of ayurveda in simple, down-to-earth language and gently coaxes the reader through a series of lifestyle changes which are guaranteed to change his or her life – in the nicest possible way. Although it is straightforward, it does not serve up a diluted, half-hearted ayurveda. It goes beyond most of the books currently available, delving into fascinating areas such as nature therapy, gem therapy, and music therapy – presenting esoteric ideas in an easily understood format. How you use this book is up to you. You can simply dip in where you choose and adopt whichever strategies you fancy, or you can work through it thoroughly, taking on board as much or little as you please. Even if you shift just one aspect of your life – make one small change – you will be setting up a chain reaction in your body and mind that will coax you towards better health.

Of course, the more shifts you make, the more profound the healing you can expect and the larger the shift towards total health and total well-being. It's up to you. But take it slowly and with thought. There's no point in forcing yourself into major changes if you are not ready – your good intentions will fade away if they don't fit in with your lifestyle. Fortunately, most of ayurveda is so practical, so straightforward, that you should not have difficulty incorporating it into your everyday life.

HISTORY AND PHILOSOPHY

This book is ultimately practical in its approach – I don't want to bog you down with pages of theory. However, it's useful (and fascinating) to know the roots of ayurveda and its prevailing philosophy. If you want to skip this part, that's fine – just head for the first chapter and wade right in.

As I've already said, ayurveda is the oldest system of medicine on earth. The ancient texts call it "eternal" as it was simply always there, always around. Its principles were said to have been passed down to humankind from a chain of gods leading back to Brahma, father of all gods. Ayurveda is generally accepted to be the forerunner of all the great healing systems of the world and written texts show that the ayurvedic medicine practiced from about 1500BC to AD500 was incredibly advanced and included detailed knowledge of pediatrics, psychiatry, surgery, geriatrics, toxicology, general medicine, and other specialties. Students studied six philosophical systems: logic, evolution and causality, the discipline of body and spirit (yoga), moral behavior, pure esoteric knowledge, and even the theory of the atom. No modern medical student would have had so thorough a grounding in such a broad spectrum of disciplines.

Historians of the ancient world wrote of the great universities which taught ayurveda. However, when India started to suffer invasions in the Middle Ages, the system began to fall apart and the universities were eventually broken up. The British almost succeeded in putting the final nail in the coffin of ayurveda by introducing their own brand of modern Western medicine and establishing their own universities. Ayurveda was in danger of dying out altogether. Fortunately, India realized what it was losing and the Indian

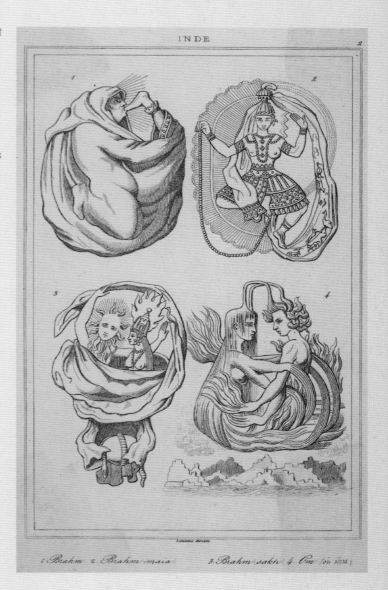

INDE

1 Brahm. 2 Brahm-maia. 3 Brahm-sakti. 4 Om (ou AUM)

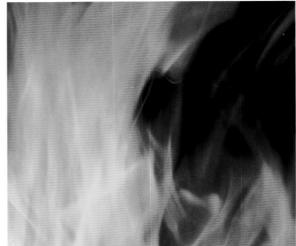

Congress affirmed its support for ayurveda. In 1921
Mahatma Gandhi opened the first new college for ayurvedic
medicine and today, in India, ayurveda is being practiced
alongside Western medicine.

Ayurvedic philosophy is incredibly complex and takes
years of study to begin to comprehend. Ayus means life,
which, in the ancient scriptures, is defined as the combination
of body, mind, and soul. In ayurveda there is no split
between body and mind – they are seen as completely
inseparable, with each influencing the other. Together they
form the physical part of a being. Yet the body-mind unit
cannot exist without soul. Soul is substance-less,
indestructible, eternal – a form of energy which animates
the body-mind.

Each person's individual soul-energy is linked with the
wider energies of the universal soul and cosmic energy. So
each of us has our own eternal life energy which is like a
spark from the universal fire – we are separate yet part of
the whole, linked with other people, and linked with the

universe. There really is no division between us and the
outer world.

In this, ayurveda pre-empts much of the new thinking in
physics, in quantum theory. Quantum physicists teach that
there is really no division between us and the world around
us: everything is made up of energy vibrating at different
speeds. They further believe that divisions of time and space
are spurious too: what happens on the other side of the
world can affect us thousands of miles away. Even more
intriguing is the idea that our role as observers is an
essential one – some even go so far as to say that the world
only exists because we are here looking at it! This also gives
a logical base for many of ayurveda's more bizarre sounding
practices. Because our energy is linked with that of the
world around us, it makes perfect sense that we should
seek harmony with our families and friends, with society, with
nature, with our environment, with the cosmos, and with the
world of spirit. It's not enough to make changes purely on
the physical or biochemical level – health and well-being

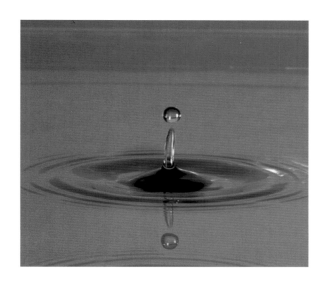 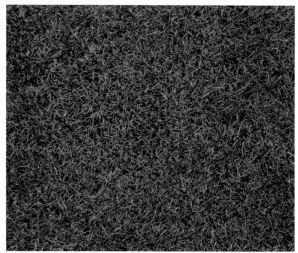

come about by achieving harmony both within ourselves and within our environment, both near and far. We need to learn how to observe and balance our own rhythms with those of nature and the wider cosmos. In this, ayurveda really is a way of life. We are taught to see ourselves as a whole and as inextricably linked with the world around us. Ayurveda is holistic in the true sense of the word.

The vedic texts teach that behind the world and cosmos as we know it, lies a state of pure consciousness, total harmony, complete awareness. It is beyond all limitations of time and space, without beginning or end. As with many world philosophies, it was considered to be the desire for pure being to experience itself which led to a split into primordial universal energy (known as purusa) and cosmic substance (prakruti). Purusa is active and energizing; it breathes life into prakruti, bringing about three essential qualities, or gunas. These are called sattva, rajas, and tamas. Sattva consists of truth, virtue, beauty, and equilibrium; rajas brings about force and impetus; while

tamas is the force of restriction and obstruction. Sattva rules our subjective world – how we perceive matter and the world around us. Tamas is the objective world, which comprises the five elements. Rajas, the force and energy of movement, brings the objective and subjective worlds together.

Let's take a closer look at tamas, the guna which makes up the world around us. On a subtle energy level, tamas consists of five subtle elements or senses – sight, sound, touch, taste, smell. These elements give rise to the dense elements – ether, air, fire, water, and earth – from which the physical world around us is born.

Put at its simplest, each physical atom consists of the five elements: its weight comes from earth, its cohesion from water, its energy from fire, its motion from air, and the space between its particles is made of ether. So the whole human body is composed of the five elements and an excess or lack of one or more elements can be the cause of imbalance and hence lead to illness.

THE THREE DOSHAS – YOUR ESSENTIAL TYPE

This may sound very complicated (and believe me, this is a much simplified version of the philosophy) but don't worry too much if you find it hard to follow. Fortunately, over the centuries, ayurveda came up with a kind of shorthand for working out imbalances – the three doshas or bio-energies, which are combinations of the five elements. Vata is a combination of ether and air, pitta of fire with water, and kapha of water and earth. In an ideal state, we would have all three doshas in perfect balance but this is rare. Most of us have one or perhaps two which overbalance the others. The whole aim of ayurvedic medicine is to balance the doshas to restore health.

Your predominating dosha can be detected by a series of physical and emotional characteristics. For example, vata people are usually thin, agile, quick-thinking, and restless; pitta people tend to be of medium build, are competitive, and make good leaders; kapha people are larger framed and more placid in nature, with great reserves of strength and endurance (you'll find out which is your predominating dosha in Part One). The aim of ayurveda is to coax all the elements into perfect balance so perfect health can follow. However complex the theory, the advice is very practical and down-to-earth. Ayurveda seeks to balance the body, using primarily a combination of lifestyle advice, diet, exercise, and herbal medicine. Massage, manipulation, marma therapy (very similar to acupressure), aromatherapy, and sound therapy are also used. Yoga, meditation, and deep breathing are highly recommended.

There is little doubt that ayurveda can achieve wonderful (some say miraculous) results. At present, research projects are trying to discover how the cures work and are investigating the properties of several ayurvedic herbs and herbal preparations. Preliminary studies by the US National Cancer Institute research project indicate that one herb, semicarpus anacardium, may inhibit the growth of certain cancers. Meanwhile, a compound of herbs called Maharishi Amrit Kalash has been found to have anticarcinogenic and antineoplastic properties – it appears to both prevent the start of cancer and decrease the size of existing tumors. A series of experiments conducted at South Dakota State University and the Ohio State University College of Medicine indicate that the compound "may have great value in the prevention and treatment of cancer."

WHAT CAN AYURVEDA TREAT?

The advice in this book will help you make changes to enhance your health and well-being but it is beyond its scope to offer advice on treating more serious health problems. However, ayurveda can and does have excellent results in dealing with chronic health problems. You may find that, by following the suggestions in this book, many niggling complaints disappear of their own accord. Without doubt you should find your digestion improve, your sleep become deeper and more restful, and your body become more supple and relaxed.

On an emotional level, you should feel calmer yet more alert and therefore better able to concentrate and more able to cope with stress.

If you want to go further, you should seek out a well-qualified ayurvedic physician (many are trained in orthodox Western medicine as well as ayurveda).

Under professional guidance the following conditions have responded well to ayurveda:

- Digestive problems: stomach ulcers, chronic gastritis, acid indigestion, heartburn, constipation, flatulence

- Gynecological problems: menstrual and menopausal difficulties

- Weight problems: weight loss and weight gain

- Skin complaints: eczema, dermatitis, psoriasis, acne

- Allergic conditions: asthma, hay fever, sinus problems

- Joint and muscle problems: chronic pain, muscle tension, sciatica, rheumatism, arthritis, osteoporosis

- Psychosomatic illness: sleep disturbances, migraine and tension headaches, depression, anxiety attacks

- Heart and circulatory problems: angina, high blood pressure, palpitations, irregular pulse

- Addictions: alcohol, smoking, drugs

- Some physicians have also treated conditions such as cancer, MS, and ME with success – and there is research into HIV/AIDS.

WHO PRACTICES AYURVEDA?

There are three categories of ayurvedic practitioners. Some have undergone a rigorous medical training for five or six years in India or Sri Lanka and are awarded degrees in Ayurvedic Medicine and Surgery – they have the letters BAMS or DAMS after their names. There are also many Western-trained healthcare practitioners (both orthodox and complementary) who incorporate ayurvedic principles into their practices. There is no means of assessing or accrediting such trainings. The third type of ayurvedic practitioner is one who offers lifestyle guidance using ayurvedic principles. They do not offer medical advice but teach how to use the principles of ayurveda in everyday life. Practitioners from all three categories can be very helpful. If at all possible, you should be guided by personal recommendation. If that's not possible, I have listed resources at the back of the book to help you find an ayurvedic professional.

1

becoming aware of body,
mind, and soul

CHAPTER ONE

building awareness

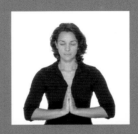

How many of us even try to understand what our bodies want and need – let alone listen to the wisdom of our unconscious minds? We're missing out. By learning how to pay attention to the many signs and signals from our bodies and inner selves, we can start a dialogue which will pay huge dividends. In ancient India, self-awareness was a vital lesson – and one that was learned at a young age. We may have a long way to go to catch up but hopefully the exercises in this chapter will swiftly start a conversation going!

Ayurveda is a holistic system in which every aspect of life becomes vitally important: from what you eat and drink, to how you think and feel. It teaches that everything in life is interconnected – if your mind is sluggish, it will affect your body. If you are full of hate, that energy will slowly and surely transform your body and distort your mind. It follows then that before we even begin to work with the wisdom of ayurveda we need to learn how to become aware. The vast majority of us spend our lives in a fog. We drift through the days barely conscious of how we feel – in our bodies, our minds, our souls. Yet once we start to listen, we soon discover that our bodies and minds are desperately trying to communicate. Try this...

BODY AWARENESS

How do you feel right now, at this very moment? Become conscious first of all of your body.

- How are you sitting? Are you slumped on a sofa or squeezed on a chair? Are you comfortable, really comfortable? Shift around a bit – notice how you feel. Would you feel better in a different position: on the floor, on a different chair, lying down? What does your body want?

- Take a journey through your body, starting with your head and neck. Is there any tension in your neck? Are you clenching your jaw? We all hold stress in our bodies but often become so used to it that we barely notice it.

- Move down through your shoulders (more tension?) to your spine and then your buttocks. How are you sitting? Is your spine straight or slumped?

- Move through your arms to your hands. How do they feel? What words pop into your head? Often our bodies know things our conscious minds don't – be open to listening to your body.

- Follow down through your thighs, knees, ankles, feet. Are your feet solidly on the ground or floating in air? Does that say anything about your attitude to life? Are you grounded or do you feel as though you live totally "in your head?"

Whenever you remember, make time to run through your body like this, noticing any stresses or tensions. On a purely practical note, it's a great way to reduce your stress levels. On a deeper level, it's a sure-fire way to gradually become more aware of your body, your emotions, and your thoughts. And awareness is the key to ayurveda.

LINKING MIND AND BODY

Ayurveda insists that body and mind are not separate but intrinsically linked. What you put in your body will affect your mind; how you think and feel will affect your body. This is a vital principle and so I'd like to demonstrate it to you right now, at this early stage. This exercise may sound strange but just spend a few minutes trying it out. You will need a partner to experiment with.

1   Have your partner sit down in a chair and make him or herself comfortable. You might instruct them to spend a few moments just becoming aware of their breathing.

2   You now stand behind them and rest one hand on their shoulder.

3   Both of you bring your attention to the hand resting on the shoulder – how does it feel? Be aware of the pressure, the temperature, the "sense" of touch.

4   Now, after a few minutes, keep your hand in exactly the same position but take your awareness away from your hand (you might look around the room or think about something entirely different). Tell your partner when you do this.

5   Now switch over – you sit down and ask your partner to repeat the exercise.

6   Share your experiences with each other.

It's an incredibly simple exercise but most people who try it are quite astonished by the results. Generally you will find that when the awareness is taken away there is a feeling that the pressure lightens, that a sense of coolness replaces warmth (or vice versa). Some people even feel quite hurt and abandoned when the awareness goes. There is a sense that a vital connection has been lost.

The implications of this exercise are profound. It shows in a very practical way that mind affects body – in this case, someone else's body. Ayurveda teaches that we should aim for mindfulness, awareness, throughout the day. It won't be possible to manage awareness in every moment, or even a lot of moments, but by focusing on what we are doing, how we are thinking, what we are feeling, we can gradually introduce more and more mindfulness into everyday life.

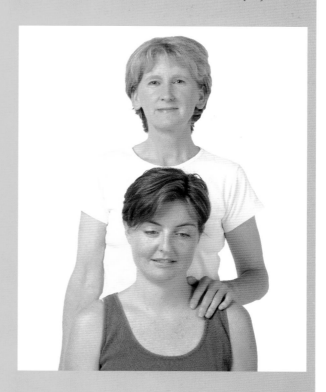

STRETCHING

As you become more familiar with ayurvedic living we will introduce hatha yoga, the ayurvedic mind-body system of exercise. But, for now, we'll start with something more familiar and close to home: simple stretching. Ayurveda teaches that in order for our bodies to function well they need to be free from tension and accumulated stress. If the body is fully stretched it allows every organ to settle comfortably into its allotted space; it also allows all the systems of the body (such as the circulation of the blood, the lymph, waste matter, hormones, and other chemicals) to move easily and in the optimum fashion. Stretching gives a workout and a wake-up call to every muscle, every ligament, every bone and tendon. Many people never bother to stretch, yet watch animals: when your dog or cat gets up after lying down it will lean forwards, bend backwards, arch its back, and stretch in a long, luxurious manner. Many yoga poses and simple stretches copy this animal wisdom: the ancient sages watched animals, copied them, and found out that they really were onto something.

So let's get stretching. Try to stretch at least once a day. Make sure your body is warm before you start. You might want to take a gentle walk outside for five or ten minutes, or march briskly on the spot for five minutes until your muscles feel warm. Follow these guidelines:

- Put your attention into the muscles you are stretching.

- Don't be tempted to "bounce" the stretch – just hold it softly.

- You should never feel pain, only a mild sense of strain. If any stretch is painful or uncomfortable it might not be for you. Be particularly careful if you have back or joint problems – check with your physician, physio, osteopath, or chiropractor before stretching.

- Breathe slowly and deeply while you stretch – it's all too easy to find yourself holding your breath, so focus on steady breathing all the time.

- Hold each stretch for a count of ten, relax, and then repeat. You should find you can stretch just that bit further.

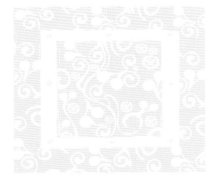

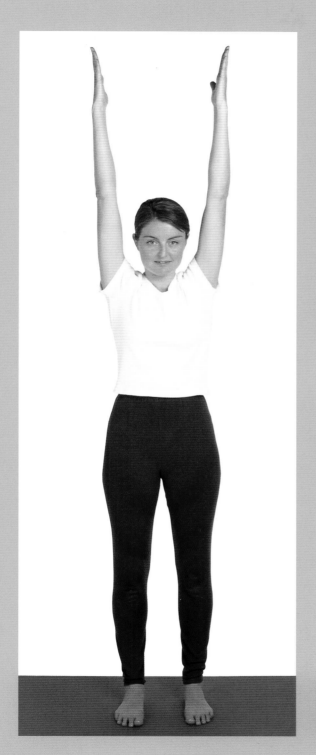

STRETCH UP TALL, SWING DOWN LOW

1   With feet shoulder-width apart and knees soft, stretch
    your arms up to the sky. Lift out of your waist, keeping
    your shoulders relaxed, and stretch up with first one
    hand, then the other. Imagine you are connecting
    yourself to the energy of the sky and heavens above.

2   Now let yourself gently flop down from the waist, letting
    your head and hands hang down towards the earth.
    Don't worry if you can't touch the floor, just hang loosely,
    imagining all the tension dropping from your body into
    the earth. Feel your feet four-square on the earth,
    grounding you and rooting you.

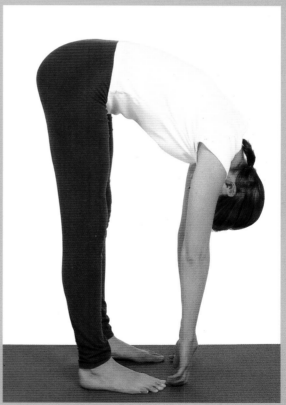

EXPAND YOUR CHEST

1 Stand with your feet shoulder-width apart, knees soft. Clasp your hands behind your back, keeping your shoulders soft and relaxed.

2 Now bring your hands away from your back until you feel a gentle stretch across your chest and across the front of your shoulders.

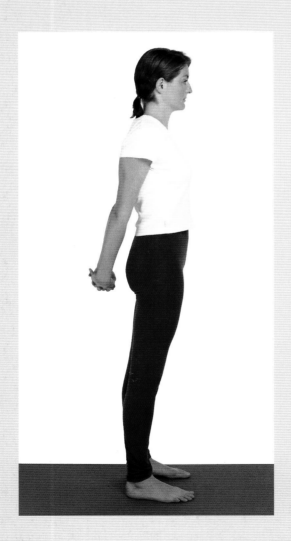

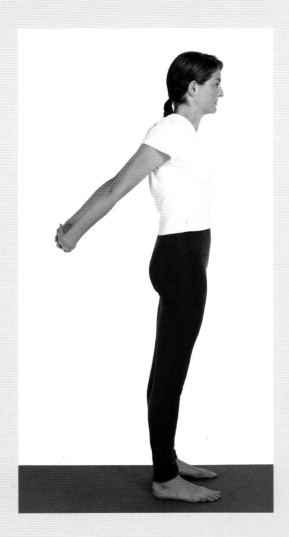

STRETCH YOUR SHOULDERS, CHEST, AND ARMS

1 Sit in an upright position or kneel – keep your shoulders relaxed and your spine straight.

2 With the back of your hand touching your spine, slide your left hand up your back (your palm will be facing outwards). Go up as far as you feel comfortable.

3 Now stretch your right arm up in the air. Bend your arm at the elbow and allow the hand to drop down your back. If you can, clasp the fingers of the other hand. If this is difficult, just go as far as you can. If you like you can use a piece of cloth – hold one end in each hand (as you become more flexible you will be able to lose the cloth). Repeat the stretch with your right hand up your back and your left hand over your shoulder.

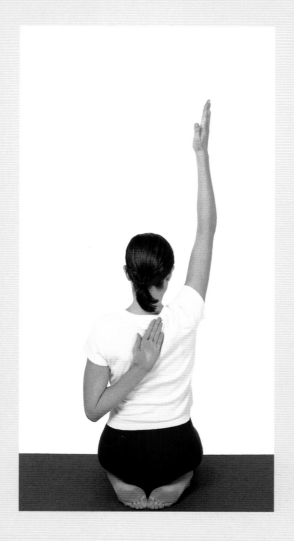

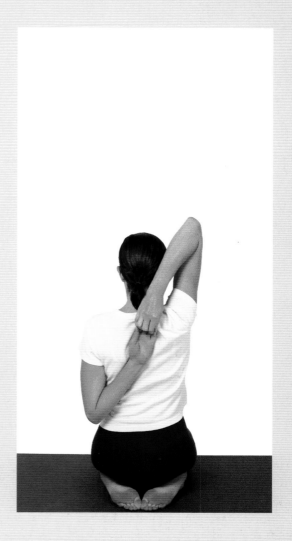

ELONGATE YOUR SPINE

1 Kneel down on the floor (make sure the floor is soft and comfortable enough – if it's hard, use a mat).

2 Stretch your body forwards over your knees until your forehead touches the floor (or moves as far as possible in that direction!)

3 Bring your arms back so they lie on the floor either side of you, then either clasp your hands behind your feet or simply stretch them along the floor towards your feet. Alternatively, bring your hands in front of your head, as if you were prostrating yourself – this version is slightly easier. Remember to breathe!

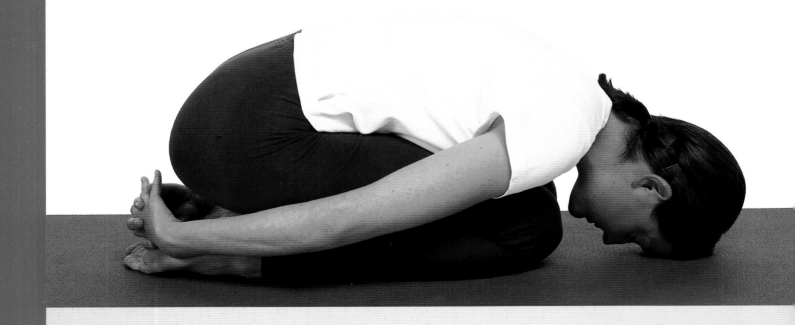

GO LONG – STRETCH STOMACH, DIAPHRAGM, AND SHOULDERS

1 Finish your stretch session by lying on the floor, on your back. Place your feet close together and point your toes. Stretch your hands over your head, fingers pointing away from your head. Tilt your pelvis slightly so you lie as flat as possible on the floor.

2 Breathe slowly and deeply. Feel your body connecting with the earth below – breathe the solidity of the earth into your body.

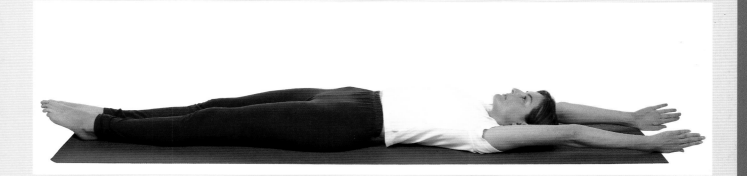

3 Close your eyes and relax. Hold for at least two minutes. Remember to breathe.

4 After this you may wish to let your toes relax, your feet flop, and your hands come gently back to your sides. Lie in this relaxed position as long as you feel comfortable – it's a good pose for assessing your body.

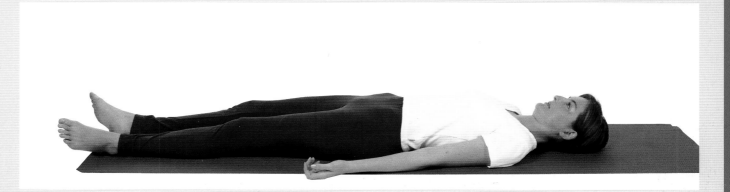

RELEASE YOUR NECK

1 Lie on your back on the floor. Tilt your pelvis up and then let it relax down to ensure your lower back is flat.

2 Slowly, very slowly, turn your head towards your right shoulder (don't let your shoulders tilt off the ground). Hold for a count of six.

3 Slowly bring your head back to center and then, again slowly, turn it towards your left shoulder. Hold here for a count of six.

4 Slowly bring it back to center and gently press your head against the floor to further release any tension in the neck.

5 Stretch your arms out sideways, at shoulder level. Bend your legs and bring your knees towards your chest.

6 Exhale and, keeping your shoulders firmly on the floor, slowly allow your knees to fall over to the left while your head slowly turns to the right.

7 Now inhale and bring your knees and head back to center.

8 Exhale and allow your knees slowly to fall over to the right while your head slowly turns to the left. Remember to keep your shoulders on the floor.

9 Inhale and bring everything back to center. Stretch out fully and breathe normally.

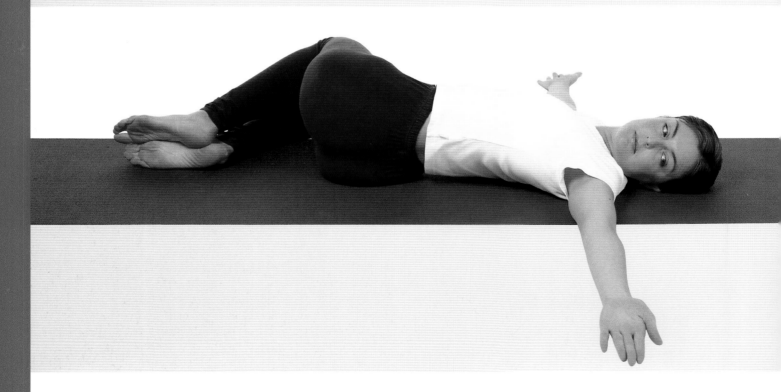

RAISING AWARENESS OF BODILY FUNCTIONS

We are a prudish bunch here in the West. We tend to divorce ourselves from the muckier, messier, smellier parts of our lives and bodies. Yet, in order to really become aware of our bodies, we need to be on intimate terms with every part of ourselves – yes, even our urine and stools! In ayurveda, every aspect of our bodies has meaning. If your urine is a different color, or has a different smell, from usual, there is a reason. If you are sweating more than usual, it might show an imbalance which needs correcting.

So start by becoming aware of your bodily functions. At this stage you don't need to worry too much about what it all means – just build awareness.

- Examine your stools. What color? What texture? Are they relatively odor-less or quite offensive? Do you evacuate regularly? Do you tend to be constipated or loose?

- Become aware of your urine. Is it clear, without much foam? Is it scanty and dull in color or strong yellow or reddish in color? Or perhaps it's very foaming.

- How much do you sweat – a lot or barely at all?

- What temperature is your body? Feel your arms and legs. Now feel your forehead – is it cooler than your arms and legs?

- Check your tongue every morning. A healthy tongue is pink with no coating. Yet many of us will find, if we bother to look, that our tongues are coated or curious variations of color.

- Look in your eyes. Again, check them every day and notice the differences – when you have had a good night's sleep and when a bad; when you have over-indulged in food and/or drink; when you are stressed and when you are relaxed.

Try to make these health checks part of your daily regimen. As you become more familiar with ayurveda you will learn that each and every one can give vital clues to which parts of you are out of balance and need attention. But over and above everything else, this awareness puts you back in touch with your body. And self-awareness is the first tool in rebuilding health.

CHAPTER TWO

which type are you?

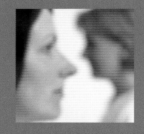

Your best friend can eat and eat yet never put on weight. You, on the other hand, only have to look at a bar of chocolate and the pounds pile on. Why? This apparent unfairness can be easily explained by ayurveda. Essentially, the answer lies in the fact that you are both governed by different energies or, as they are known in ayurvedic terms, doshas. The whole of life can be understood in terms of three forms of energy: vata (air and ether), pitta (mainly fire), and kapha (earth and water). In this chapter we'll look at this theory and how you can tell which elements are ruling (or ruining!) your life.

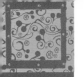

If you read the introduction, you will already know about "doshas" – if not, don't worry, we'll recap right now. Ayurveda teaches that the world and everything in it consists of five elements – earth, water, fire, air, and ether. The ancient sages even understood the concept of the atom and used this tiny block of matter to demonstrate the action of the elements. They said that the weight of the atom comes from earth, its cohesion from water, its energy from fire, its motion from air, and the spaces between its particles are made of ether. The whole human body is made up of the five elements and, according to Indian philosophy, an excess of one or more elements can be the cause of imbalance, which will eventually and inevitably lead to illness.

Over the centuries, ayurveda came up with a kind of shorthand for the five elements by combining them into three bio-energies, or "tridoshas." Some people call them "mind-body types" – we will call them doshas or types for short. These are known individually as vata, pitta, and kapha. The bio-energy, or dosha, vata comes from a combination of ether and air; pitta from fire with a little water; and kapha from water and earth. In an ideal state we would have all three doshas in perfect balance, though this is rare. Most of us have one or perhaps two which overshadow the others. The entire aim of ayurvedic medicine is to balance the doshas in order to restore health.

Each dosha is responsible for different parts and functions in the body. Vata produces movement, pitta produces heat and so is responsible for the metabolism, while kapha produces growth and structure. All three are essential for life. Without vata we couldn't breathe, blood wouldn't pump round the body, food wouldn't move through our gut, nor would any chemical impulses fly to and from the brain.

Without pitta we couldn't process the air, water, and food that runs through our system. And without kapha we simply wouldn't hold together – kapha keeps our cells bonded together and fuses bone, muscle, fat, and connective tissue.

The dosha that dominates within our body gives rise to our prakruti, or body type. This is the basic predominating psychophysiological force which affects everything about us – our shape and weight, our predisposition to different illnesses, the forms of exercise that suit us, the kinds of food we should eat, how we think, how we react to situations, even how we perceive the whole world. Ayurveda teaches that we should follow a seasonal routine to keep ourselves in balance as the seasons, and prevailing energies, change. They even have a name for the process – ritucharya. Ritucharya doesn't involve overturning your lifestyle every few months, it simply means being aware of the shifts in the seasons and moving the emphasis of your diet and activities accordingly. We'll look at this in greater detail in Part Five.

WORKING OUT YOUR PRAKRUTI

Few people have just one dosha predominating – most of us are combinations of two. If you are truly balanced already, you will be a perfect balance between all three though, as I have already said, that is quite rare. The following questionnaire should help you gain a general understanding of the doshas that govern you. Simply read through the following questions and tick those that apply to you. There are no trick questions, no right or wrong answers...just be totally and brutally honest (if you prefer you might want to write your answers on a pad).

YOUR PHYSICAL BODY

1 What were you like at birth and as a child?

a) I was small at birth and a thin child.

b) I was average at birth and a medium-sized child.

c) I was a large baby and a plump or solid child.

2 What is your build now?

a) Thin with light bones and prominent joints and tendons. Perhaps either very tall or very short, I hardly ever put on weight.

b) Medium build and bone structure, I can easily gain and lose weight.

c) Large boned and quite heavy or dense in build, with broad shoulders or wide hips. I find it hard to lose weight.

3 What is your skin like?

a) Dry, delicate skin that is easily affected by the weather.

b) Soft skin. Often a ruddy or freckled complexion.

c) Often a pale complexion with thick skin. Skin can be oily but will usually be cool to the touch.

4 What kind of hair do you have?

a) Normal to dry, often dark, wiry or kinky.

b) Normal to fine hair, often blonde, red or prematurely gray.

c) Normal to oily, thick wavy hair.

5 What are your eyes like?

a) Small, dark, and constantly moving.

b) Quite penetrating, often green, gray, or hazel.

c) Large, beautiful eyes (often brown) with lustrous eyelashes.

6 What kind of appetite do you have?

a) Irregular – sometimes I'm ravenous, sometimes I can't be bothered. I like to snack or nibble and often have eyes bigger than my stomach when it comes to large meals.

b) Good – I hate to skip meals and feel irritable and even ill if forced to do so. I like high-protein foods like meat, fish, eggs, and legumes.

c) Healthy – I enjoy food and don't like skipping meals but, if forced to do so, I suffer no ill effects. I love starchy, fatty foods such as bread, sweets, and cakes.

7 How are your bowel movements?

a) Irregular, often hard or constipated.

b) Regular, tending to soft, loose, and profuse.

c) Regular, steady, thick, and heavy.

8 How do you sleep?

a) I'm a light sleeper – sleep is often short and interrupted. I sometimes find it hard to get to sleep or I'm liable to insomnia.

b) I'm a regular and sound sleeper, and rarely have any problems.

c) I'm a heavy, long sleeper. Can be liable to oversleep or feel drowsy during the day.

9 What are your hands and nails like?

a) Cold hands with little perspiration, nails are often brittle.

b) Hands often perspire a lot, nails are flexible but quite strong.

c) Hands sometimes perspire, nails are thick and strong.

10 How do you walk?

  a) Quickly, lightly; I always seem in a hurry.

  b) Medium pace but a determined fashion; purposeful.

  c) Slowly and steadily; calm.

11 What kind of illnesses are you prone to?

  a) Sharp pains, headaches, nervous disorders, gas or constipation, eczema or dry rashes.

  b) Rashes and allergies, inflammation, heartburn, ulcers, acidity, feverish complaints.

  c) Fluid retention and excess mucus, bronchitis, sinus problems, asthma, congestion.

YOUR MIND AND EMOTIONS

12 What is your basic personality?

  a) Enthusiastic, outgoing, talkative but with changeable moods and ideas.

  b) Strong-minded and purposeful, I thrive on challenges. I tend to be quite forceful in expressing my opinions.

  c) Calm and can be placid and good-natured, easy-going, reliable, and steady.

13 What are you like at work?

  a) Quick, imaginative, and alert; an active and creative thinker with an endless fund of ideas. I become bored with rigid routine or discipline.

  b) A natural leader with a keen intellect. I'm efficient, like well-planned routine, and tend to be a perfectionist.

  c) I keep projects running smoothly and calmly. I enjoy a regular routine.

14 How do you react to stress?

  a) I have a tendency to become anxious or nervous.

  b) I become angry or irritable.

  c) I try to avoid it at all costs.

15 How do you dream?

  a) Frequently but I often can't remember my dreams on waking.

  b) Vividly, often in color – I find it easy to remember my dreams.

  c) I only tend to remember highly significant or clear dreams.

16 How is your sex life?

  a) I have an active fantasy life but my sexual interest tends to fluctuate.

  b) I have a pretty average sex drive.

  c) I love sex and although I might take a while to "warm up," I have intense sex and great stamina.

17 Do you spend or save money?

  a) Money is there to spend; I tend to be an impulse-buyer and have large credit-card bills.

  b) I am a sensible spender, buying useful and classic items.

  c) I am a great saver, I always have enough money.

18 How would you describe your lifestyle?

  a) Erratic, always changing.

  b) Busy with plenty of plans; I achieve a lot.

  c) Steady and regular; I sometimes feel a bit stuck in a rut.

Now simply add up how many a's, b's, and c's you ticked.

A predominance of a's indicate vata.

A predominance of b's indicate pitta.

A predominance of c's indicate kapha.

Few people ever have just one dosha so don't be surprised if you have two scores quite close. Most of us are combinations of two doshas – some people even have all three. Let's have a quick look at what your scores mean.

Mainly A's – VATA

Speed and movement are the keys to vata, so it's not surprising to find that vata is the dosha of wind and air. If you're a typical vata you are always on the go, both physically and mentally. Vatas are quick, creative, and flexible; they absolutely adore anything new and exciting – new things, new ideas, new sights. Vatas are ideas people, full of imagination and often artistic. However, it is hard to pin them down to one task or one idea; they are changeable and tend to flit from one thing to another. Vatas pick up new subjects very quickly and easily but often forget them just as quickly.

Times dominated by vata energy: Vata energy is most active in the late afternoon and early evening (from 2–6pm) and just before dawn (2–6am). Its seasons are fall and winter.

When vata is unbalanced: When vata is unbalanced it can cause constipation, bloating and wind, aching joints, dry skin and hair, brittle nails, failing memory or confusion.

Mainly B's – PITTA

Fire and water are the elements of pitta. If you're a pitta person you will undoubtedly have initiative and good energy; you are a determined and forceful soul, confident in your abilities, courageous, intelligent, and generally happy. Pittas grasp information quickly and easily and can put their knowledge into practice. They are great organizers in whatever field they find themselves – either as highly organized parents or the leaders of large corporations.

Times dominated by pitta energy: Pitta energy is strongest between 10am and 2pm and from 10pm to 2am. Its season is high summer.

When pitta is unbalanced: If pitta energy becomes unbalanced you can fall prey to sunburn, rashes, and irritability in the sun. Sore throats, inflammations, and fevers, and intense feelings of anger, frustration, or jealousy are all signs of unbalanced pitta.

Mainly C's – KAPHA

Solidity is the key word for kapha, the dosha of earth and water. Kapha is solid, strong, and enduring, and if you're a kapha person you're probably as "strong as an ox" with great stamina. Kaphas are wonderfully calm, grounded, honest, and trustworthy people who prefer to shun the limelight and quietly work on the task in hand. Kapha people crave security; they enjoy routines and the comforts of regularity. They most definitely like their food and can often comfort eat and put on weight.

Times dominated by kapha energy: Kapha times are 6–10am and 6–10pm. The kapha season is spring.

When kapha is unbalanced: When kapha falls into imbalance, you will find excess weight and mucus building in the body, sinuses will become blocked, and colds will become common. Depression is the bane of unbalanced kapha.

Finding and balancing your doshas can be a truly liberating experience. People who have never been able to lose weight, for example, can find the excess simply vanishing as they rid their body of the foods that increase kapha dosha. The benefits aren't just physical: soothing imbalanced doshas can help your memory and concentration, can allow you to sleep better, can help you deal with stress, make you less irritable, and even improve your sex life.

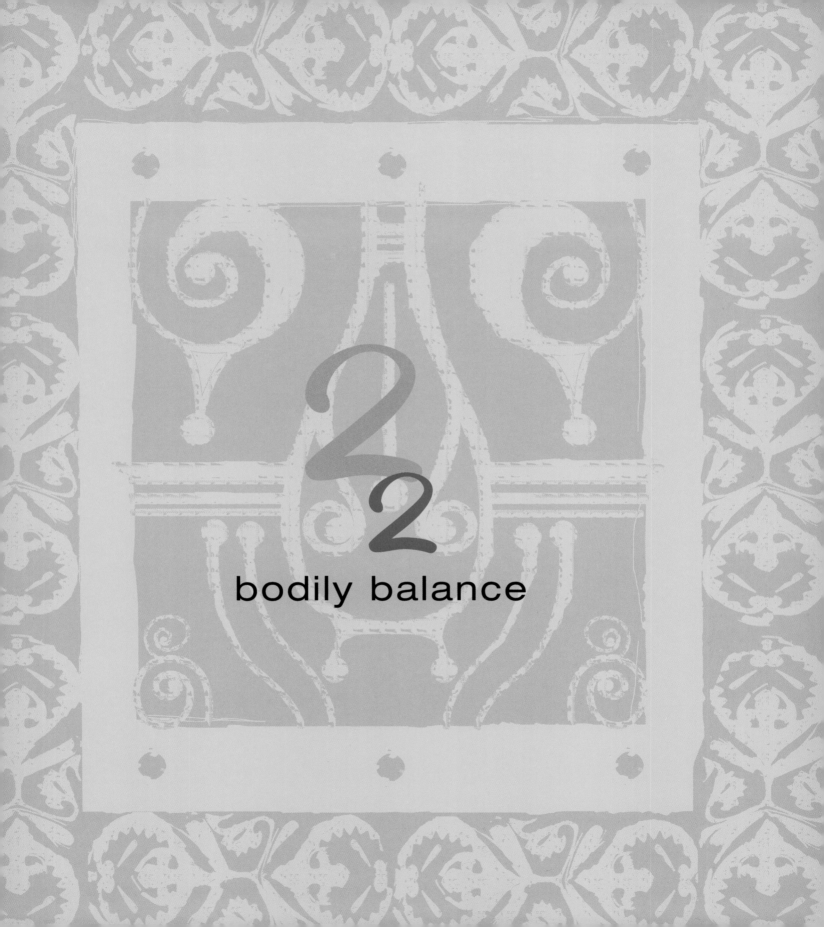

2
2
bodily balance

CHAPTER THREE

first steps in transforming your life

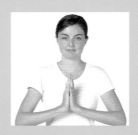

Now you know which dosha is predominant in your life, you can start to use this information in a highly practical way. In ayurveda even the tiniest shifts and changes can make an enormous difference and most physicians will use lifestyle changes before any more drastic therapies. In this chapter we're going to look at how you can balance and soothe any energies which are out of kilter – often using quite unexpected diagnosis and techniques!

The beauty of ayurveda is that you don't need to change your entire lifestyle all in one fell swoop. Even small shifts will have great effects and, as you notice your health and well-being improving, you will most probably be motivated to introduce more changes.

Throughout the book we will be looking at subtle and simple ways to change your life. But let's start with something dramatic. One of the swiftest ways to bring about positive change is to make changes which will calm your predominant dosha. As we've already discussed, we all have within us the three energies or doshas – vata, pitta, and kapha. One or two will predominate and "rule" our bodies and minds. However, modern living takes a profound toll on us and it is incredibly easy for one or more doshas to

FINDING IMBALANCES

The following short questionnaire should give you an idea in which dosha you have an imbalance. Once again simply tick the questions that you can answer "yes" to. If you have several ticks in any category it is quite likely that you have an imbalance in that dosha.

VATA IMBALANCE

1 Are you seriously underweight?
2 Do you have eczema or dry, rough, chapped skin?
3 Do you suffer from constipation or bad wind?
4 Do you find it hard to concentrate, difficult to relax? Do you constantly jump up to do things?
5 Is your sleep very disturbed? Do you find it hard to get to sleep or have bad insomnia?
6 Are your hands and feet often cold? Do you have bad circulation?
7 Do you often have headaches or migraines?
8 Are you constantly overexerting yourself?

fall out of balance. When this happens, we start to feel unwell, off color, irritable, tired, and generally out of sorts. Yet there are very simple steps you can take to soothe an unbalanced dosha and coax it back into a state of peace. Of course, if you possibly can, it's best to see a professional ayurvedic physician – but there's also plenty we can do for ourselves. The advice that follows in this chapter offers simple first steps to soothe your doshas.

At this point many people become slightly confused. If you have two prevailing doshas, which should you soothe? One way is to check to see which dosha has the major imbalance.

PITTA IMBALANCE

1   Do you suffer from heartburn, ulcers, or acidity?
2   Are you frequently irritable, impatient, and critical?
3   Are you over-ambitious, too demanding, and stubborn?
4   If you are stressed, do you tend to overreact and get angry or frustrated?
5   Do you break out in rashes easily? Are you very susceptible to bad food or unpleasant environmental pollution?
6   Do you often have diarrhea?
7   Do you often get feverish colds and flus?
8   Do you react badly to the heat and sun?

KAPHA IMBALANCE

1   Is your skin dull and congested with enlarged pores?
2   Are you very overweight and finding it impossible to shift?
3   Do you become possessive and over-attached to people and things?
4   Do you feel uncomfortable in cool, damp weather?
5   Do you have a lot of mucus or related problems such as blocked sinuses, asthma, bronchitis, or phlegm?
6   Are you very lethargic and over-complacent? Do you lack the energy to change?
7   Do you often oversleep or find yourself dozing off during the day?
8   Are you greedy?

BODILY SIGNS AND SYMPTOMS

In ayurveda, your body really does tell the truth. If you visit an ayurvedic physician he or she will be interested in every part of your body. The major form of diagnosis is through pulse taking, which is far too complicated and subtle to teach in a book! However, there are simpler ways to listen to what your body has to say and hopefully you're now becoming more aware of your bodily functions! Let's take a moment to see what they might mean. This can be particularly useful if you're still not quite sure which dosha is unbalanced.

URINE

- Vata is disturbed if you urinate frequently but in small amounts. Your urine will be a pale yellow and thin in quality.
- Pitta is disturbed if your urine is dark yellow and strong smelling.
- Kapha is disturbed when your urine is copious, white, and foaming.

STOOLS

- Vata is disturbed if you are constipated and your stools are hard, dry, often in small "rabbit droppings." They might be gray or black in color.

- Pitta is disturbed if your stools are yellowish, blackish-yellow, or greenish in color and liquid in consistency. You may have a burning feeling as you pass the stools.
- Kapha is disturbed if your stools are whitish in color with mucus or undigested food.

TONGUE

- Over-abundant vata is likely if your tongue is dry, cool, and rough to the touch. There may be a reddish-brown coating. You may also notice a sweet taste in your mouth.
- Disturbed pitta is often indicated when the tongue is dark red or has a yellowish coating. It may feel soft and slimy and you might have a persistent bitter, sharp taste in the mouth.
- Disturbed kapha is likely when there is a lot of saliva in the mouth. The tongue may feel sticky and rough and there may be a white coating. If there is a taste present it is usually sweet and salty.

SKIN

- Vata is disturbed when the skin feels rough and dry.
- Pitta is disturbed when the skin feels hot to the touch.
- Kapha is disturbed when the body perspires and the skin feels sticky.

There are plenty of other ways of observing imbalance in the body but I think this is quite sufficient for beginners!

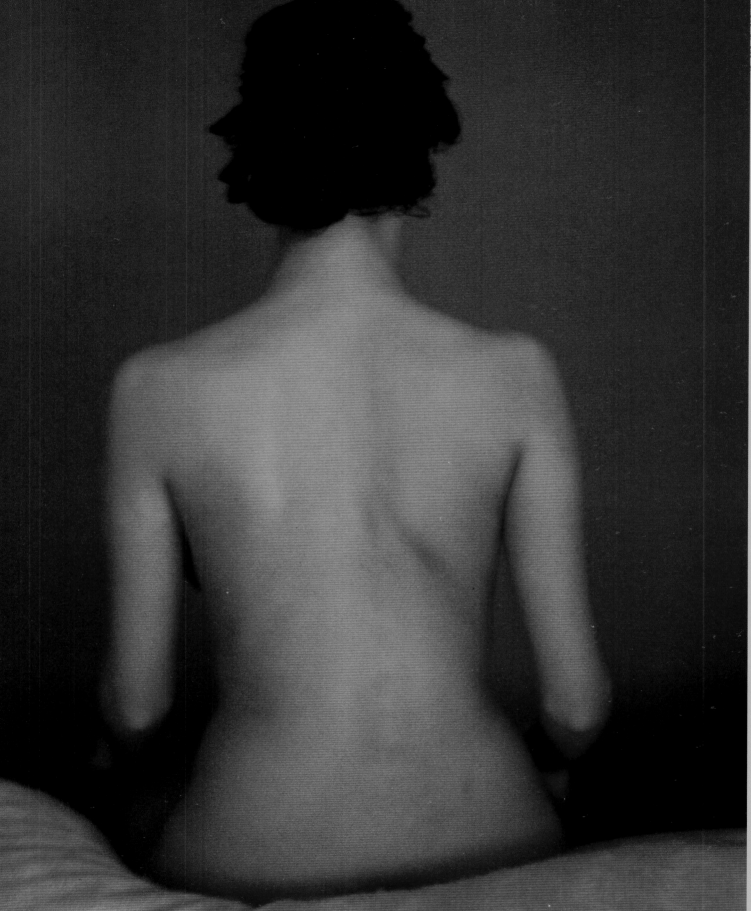

BALANCING PITTA

Follow these guidelines if you are predominantly pitta or have a pitta imbalance.

- Keep your cool – in all ways. Avoid the physical heat: stay out of the hot sun and keep clear of steams and saunas (although you probably love them) as they combine heat and humidity, the two things you need to shun. If you have a warm bath or shower, finish off with a cool rinse. Get out in the open air as much as you can, but if it's hot keep cool in the shade.

- Pittas are usually highly organized; in fact, remarkably organized. Maybe you need to introduce a little spontaneity into your life. Be careful that you don't become too goal-orientated; too focused on objectives and nothing else. Try taking a walk "for the hell of it." Lounging in the garden or gazing out of the window – not doing anything in particular, just musing, is highly therapeutic for pittas.

- If you're a typical pitta you thrive on challenge, hate being bored, and love a little competition in life.

Obviously you shouldn't get bored, but don't take on too much or challenge yourself too far. Be careful that you don't end up sacrificing everything just to win.

- Pittas are naturals in competitive sports such as tennis and squash, and even an innocent game of ping-pong can bring out the killer serve. They can easily take sport far too seriously and if you know you're a pitta type you should avoid anything too competitive. Water sports are wonderfully calming and soothing for pitta – and, of course, winter sports in the snow and ice will cool that pitta fire.

- Pittas love hot spicy foods, meat, and alcohol (they are the stereotypical curry and beer, or steak and red-wine-drinking business types) but such meals are their absolute bane. It may be difficult but you need to avoid (or at the very least cut right down) oily or greasy foods, caffeine, salt, red meat, alcohol, and any highly-spiced foods. Foods that tend to cool and calm pitta include fresh fruit and vegetables, milk, soft cheeses (not hard cheese), cottage cheese, and ice cream. Wholegrains are fine for pitta and greens provide the bitter taste that can balance pitta so well.

BALANCING KAPHA

Follow these guidelines if you are predominantly kapha or have a kapha imbalance.

- Learn to let go. Kaphas hoard, they hang onto things like grim death – be it weight, people, or emotions. If you're a kapha, loosen up, trust a little, release, let go – there is more, you know, you won't be left lacking!

- Get out of your rut: allow change, unpredictability, and excitement into your life. Kaphas feel snug, safe, and secure when everything stays the same but taking the odd chance or allowing the pulse rate to speed up a little from time to time will give any sluggish kapha energy a good boost. You don't have to bet your home on a turn of the dice, even little things can help – vary your route to work; shift the furniture round in your office or home; if you always have a drink at 6pm, go for a walk instead...

- Kaphas love to sit around doing nothing in particular. They are champions at the fine art of staring into space. To balance kapha, you need to get your system moving, give it a bit of a shake-up. You want activities that will stimulate you both physically and mentally, so take on new activities and challenges – try a new sport or a night class or watch different types of films or television shows. Keep your activities varied – if you do aerobics, try step or kickboxing; if you do circuits, try a long distance run. If you don't do anything (except walking from the car to the take-out) do something, anything. Kaphas need plenty of physical exercise – try to incorporate some activity into every day.

- On vacation, kaphas are the ones who slide into a sun-lounger in the morning and have to be peeled off it in the evening. To stimulate kapha, go on a touring vacation or challenge yourself to an activity break where you will have constant stimulation.

- Avoid iced food and drink, cut right down on candy, and don't eat too much bread. Dairy produce will aggravate kapha – it produces yet more mucus – and wheat can often be a problem too. Heavy starchy foods are really unsuitable for kapha. Instead eat warm, light, and dry foods – nothing stodgy or greasy. However, kapha does need a certain amount of complex carbohydrate to function well – try using grains such as millet, barley, and rye which are all light and dry. Plenty of fresh vegetables will help, and use herbs and spices liberally.

CHAPTER FOUR

eat for health and vitality

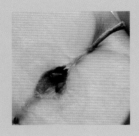

If you're yearning for good health, vitality, and a sense of calm and focus, look to your diet. The old adage "we are what we eat" is quite true and in India food is used as vital medicine. It's not just what you eat (although that is certainly important), it's also how you eat it. Ayurveda has a host of rules for good eating which are not only intensely practical but which also make good nutritional and digestive sense. It's certainly not hair-shirt draconian dieting either: ayurveda teaches that food and eating should, above all, be enjoyable.

Diet is the basis of good health. Eat well and you will feel good – it's often as simple as that. Unfortunately most of us in the West have lousy nutrition. We eat diets clogged with fat, sugar, and refined food. We tend to eat "on the run" or for convenience, choking our systems with junk food, fast food, or "ready" meals that someone else has prepared for us. Such foods are not fuel for the body and mind – they provide calories but not true energy. In ayurveda, food is medicine. Eat correctly – choose the right foods, prepare them properly, eat mindfully – and a host of ailments will clear up. You should feel brighter and happier and your body will undoubtedly be healthier.

The ayurvedic philosophy of food is very complex, too complex for the pages of this book. Most of the practice, however, is very simple. Let's start with some general principles...

THE TEN RULES OF HEALTHY EATING

1   Set aside enough time to prepare and eat your food. Eat in a calm, pleasant atmosphere and concentrate on what you're eating – don't read a book or watch television. Always sit down to eat.

2   Choose foods which are attractive and wholesome, both to your taste buds and your eyes. Prepare your table with care too: a fresh tablecloth and flowers, perhaps some candles.

3   Try to eat at the same time each day. Be mindful of what you eat and be aware of your appetite – stop when you are not quite full. Never eat to excess. Eat your food slowly and chew each mouthful thoroughly, paying attention to the texture and taste of the food.

4   Always make sure you have digested your last meal before eating another. Generally you should allow three to six hours between meals. Don't eat if you are not hungry.

5   Avoid ice-cold drinks, particularly around and with meals. Drink hot water with your meals (this takes a little getting used to but is quite pleasant). If you want to take cold drinks (or ice cream or sorbets) eat them in-between meals, or warm your stomach with a cup of ginger tea beforehand.

6   Choose your food with care. Ideally the bulk (if not all) of your diet should come from organic, locally-produced, seasonal food. The majority of your meal should consist of warm, freshly-prepared food which is easy to digest. Avoid re-heated or leftover food – it is considered "dead" food.

7   Make lunch, the midday meal, the main meal of the day. Your digestion functions best between noon and 1pm.

8   The digestive fire, known as agni, is low by evening – so make this meal small and easily digested. Avoid serving heavy dairy produce, animal protein, and raw, cold foods at this meal.

9   Don't race up after your meal. Allow yourself a few minutes of calm relaxation. Relax, sit quietly, and give thanks for your food. Take a gentle walk, if you can, to aid digestion.

10 Notice how you feel after each meal. Become aware of what foods your body likes and doesn't like. What do certain foods do for your energy levels? Do any make your heart race or make you feel breathless, uncomfortable, or bloated? Start to be guided by your body when it comes to your food choices.

DIET AND THE DOSHAS

Food is one of the prime ways we can balance the doshas. In an ideal world we would all be so in touch with our bodies and their needs that we would automatically eat the correct foods. Unfortunately, we have become so divorced from our natural processes that few of us really listen and understand our bodies. The best course of action then is to choose a diet rich in foods which balance or soothe your main dosha.

FOODS TO SOOTHE VATA

People who are predominantly vata or have strong vata imbalance should ensure that, above all, they eat at regular times in a calm, relaxed atmosphere. Their diet should be warming and nourishing with plenty of salty, sour, and sweet tastes. So boost the following in your diet:

- dairy produce – milk, cream, cheese, butter, yogurt, ghee (clarified butter)
- natural sweeteners – honey, cane sugar, maple syrup
- all types of nuts and seeds, but in small amounts
- chicken, duck, fish, seafood
- eggs
- sesame oil
- wheat and rice, cooked oats
- sweet, ripe fruits such as bananas, apricots, mango, melon, pineapple, papaya, peaches, berries, figs etc.
- vegetables cooked with a little added ghee – garlic and onions, asparagus, beet/beetroot, carrots, cucumber, sweet potato, green beans
- pulses: red lentils, mung dal, urad dal
- herbs: those with sweet and warming tastes such as basil, marjoram, cilantro/coriander, fennel, bay leaves, oregano, sage, tarragon, thyme
- spices: again, warming sweet spices such as licorice, mace, caraway, cardamom, cinnamon, cloves, cumin, ginger, mustard, black pepper, nutmeg

VATA should avoid the following:

- raw vegetables and salads, cabbage, cauliflower, sweet peppers, mushrooms, bean sprouts
- dried fruits, unripe fruit (particularly bananas), cranberries, pears, pomegranate
- millet, maize, barley, buckwheat, rye, uncooked oats
- all pulses aside from those mentioned above
- lamb, pork, game
- white sugar

FOODS TO SOOTHE PITTA

Pitta is hot and so people with pitta predominant or out of balance need to cool themselves down. Anything that makes you hot – such as salt, hot pungent spices, seasonings, oil – should be avoided. Bitter and astringent tastes are useful for pitta. Pittas should aim for calm mealtimes too – often stress causes them to miss meals or eat on the hoof.

These are the foods which suit pitta particularly well:

- unsalted butter, ghee, milk, ice cream, cottage cheese
- almost all kinds of pulses and legumes, except those given below
- barley, cooked oats, wheat, white rice
- poultry, rabbit, fish (freshwater, in moderation)
- egg (but just the whites)
- fruit juice concentrates and maple syrup
- vegetables: asparagus, cucumber, broccoli, Brussels sprouts, cabbage, celery, green beans, all green leafy vegetables, mushrooms, potatoes, sweet peppers, zucchini/courgettes, bean sprouts, chicory
- ripe and sweet fruits: apples, coconut, figs, grapes, mango, cherries (but must be sweet), raisins, prunes, oranges
- sunflower and pumpkin seeds
- spices: cardamom, cinnamon, saffron, turmeric, ginger, black pepper (in small amounts)
- herbs: dill, fennel, mint

PITTA should avoid the following:

- all sour milk products, such as yogurt, hard cheese, buttermilk, sour cream
- all sour fruits
- corn, millet, maize, buckwheat, rye, brown rice
- almond, sesame, and corn oils
- sesame seeds
- all nuts (except coconut and soaked and peeled almonds)
- red meat, all seafood, venison
- egg yolks
- beet/beetroot, eggplant/aubergine, radish, tomatoes, chili peppers, spinach, onions
- all hot spices such as cayenne, chili, aniseed, cloves, mustard seeds
- salt, vinegar, pickles, ketchups, and spicy sauces

FOODS TO SOOTHE KAPHA

Kapha should aim for a light, dry, and hot diet. Anything heavy, fatty, or cold will weigh kapha down and make you sluggish and more prone than usual to putting on weight (a perennial kapha problem). Aim for low-fat, spicy, lightly-cooked meals.

These foods will help balance your constitution:

- skimmed goat's milk, buttermilk, ghee (in small quantities)
- all pulses except those listed below
- poultry, shrimp, game (in small seasonal quantities)
- sunflower and pumpkin seeds
- raw honey
- small amounts of oils and fat: ghee, almond oil, corn, sunflower oil
- barley, buckwheat, corn, maize, millet, rye
- most vegetables – see below for the exceptions
- fruit: apples, pears, pomegranate, cranberries, figs, dried fruits
- herbs: all and plenty
- spices: all and plenty, especially ginger, black pepper, coriander, turmeric, cloves, cardamom, cinnamon

KAPHA should avoid the following:

- cucumber, sweet potatoes, zucchini/courgettes, pumpkin, squash
- bananas, grapes, melon, plums, mango, coconut
- cheese, yogurt, sour milk, cream, full-fat milk, butter, ice cream, large quantities of ghee (a little is fine)
- brown rice, oats, wheat, or white rice in large quantities
- all kinds of nuts
- sugar, molasses, syrups
- seafood (except shrimp), beef, pork, lamb, duck
- black lentils, soya beans, kidney beans
- salt

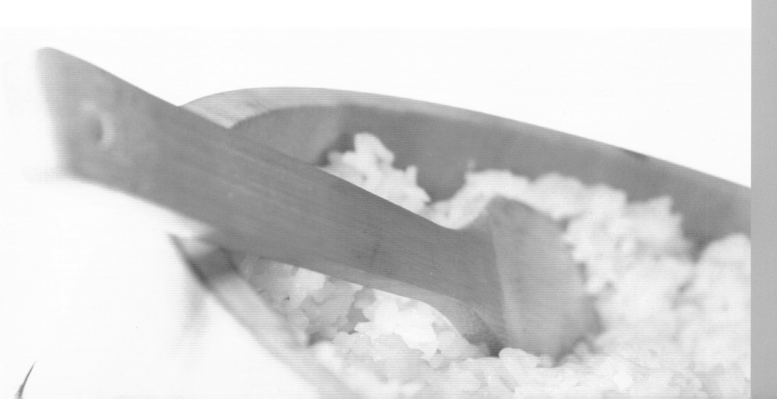

If you start to shift your diet towards one which supports your leading dosha you should soon notice you start to feel better. If you have problems with your weight, whether you're over or underweight, this should balance itself automatically when you soothe your dosha (usually vata for underweight, kapha for overweight). Before we leave this introduction to ayurvedic eating, there are just a few other pointers...

BALANCING AGNI

Agni is the name given to our digestive fire, which helps us digest and utilize the food we eat. Unfortunately, agni often becomes dampened and sluggish, or over-excited. If you have too little agni you will probably find you have a lot of gas and wind, you may be constipated, and find it tough to wake up in the morning. If, on the other hand, you have too much agni, you may belch and burp a lot, but more likely you will find you suffer from acidity – burning in the stomach or intestinal tract. You may also have diarrhea and be irritable and very thirsty. As you might suspect, this can be a result of irritated pitta, caused by eating too many hot foods or becoming overly stressed and angry.

The following measures can help to balance agni.

- Eat smaller, simpler meals.
- If agni is low, try drinking warm water to which you have added fresh lemon or lime.
- Ginger tea reduces gas and will rekindle agni.
- Adding cumin, coriander, and fennel to your meals is another way to balance agni.

THE SACRED COOKFIRE

Cooking is a magical act – it's pure alchemy. How you cook is as important as what you cook, so always bring awareness, love, and a desire to heal into your cookery.

Prana, the life force of the universe, is everywhere. Ayurveda teaches that prana can be ingested when you eat a good meal. When you cook with love, you can transfer the love you feel into the food, which will then be spread out to everyone who eats your food. Try to follow these guidelines for your cooking.

- Take care choosing your food – pick the very freshest, most local, seasonal, organic food you can find. If you eat meat, ensure it has been farmed with care and consideration for the animals. Think about perhaps growing some of your own food, even if it's just a window box with herbs.

- Say a prayer or blessing before you start. Hold your hands over your ingredients and thank them for giving their life for you. Visualize the journey of your ingredients – how they grew, who tended them, how they came to be on your table. Ask them to help nourish you and your family with love.

- Prepare your food with love and attention. Concentrate on the task at hand – look on it as sacred meditation. Try not to distract yourself by watching television or listening to the radio as you cook. Take time to notice the textures, scents, and feel of the food you are cooking. Avoid gadgets and processors where possible – hand-chopping brings you into closer contact with the food.

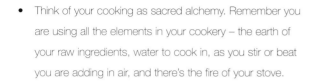

- Think of your cooking as sacred alchemy. Remember you are using all the elements in your cookery – the earth of your raw ingredients, water to cook in, as you stir or beat you are adding in air, and there's the fire of your stove.

- Pour in your hopes and wishes for the people who will eat your food as you cook. Focus your intention as you chop, stir, mix, blend. Cookery is a kind of spell-making. If you add herbs and spices with their magical properties, you can increase the power.

- Serve your meal so that it looks inviting and appetizing. Choose colors which complement each other.

- Say grace or a blessing before you eat. It need not be religious or involved – just a simple "thank-you" to the cook and the food is enough.

- Eat your food mindfully. Smell the different fragrances before you start to eat. Notice how you choose your food – be aware of putting it on your fork and in your mouth. Don't just swallow – really taste the food, feel its texture. Make each mouthful mindful.

- Clean up with mindfulness and gratitude too. Try adding a few drops of mandarin oil to your washing up liquid to cheer up your senses.

Weight Loss

If you're trying to lose weight – like a great many other people – ayurveda can help. In general you should:

⚐ Follow the guidelines for kapha eating (although not all weight problems are caused by kapha imbalance, the vast majority will respond to this regimen).

⚐ Eat your meals facing east. Your place of eating should also be calm and uncluttered.

⚐ Before you eat, chew some ginger marinated in lemon or lime juice to stimulate your digestion (if you suffer from stomach acidity you may need to omit this step).

⚐ Focus on your food – become conscious of every mouthful.

⚐ Sip nothing but warm water with your meal.

⚐ Go for a walk after your meal to help digestion.

⚐ Try to eat your largest meal at lunchtime – and don't eat after 7pm.

⚐ Practice yoga and pranayama. Stretching and deep breathing will help the weight-loss process.

CHAPTER FIVE

daily routine

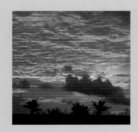

How do you structure your day? You might imagine it doesn't matter what time you get up or go to bed; when you exercise and when you eat your meals. But curiously enough, a good daily routine is the bedrock of ayurvedic healthy living. At first reading, the ideas in this chapter may sound impractical or downright insane. But do try them. After a few days you will start to notice a real dividend in terms of increased energy, better digestion, and a sounder night's sleep.

Every ayurvedic physician will prescribe a daily routine. At first it seems rather pedantic and slightly impractical – all in all, a strange approach to health. But how you live your life on a day-to-day basis is instrumental in achieving health, harmony, and happiness. Ayurveda follows the teachings of nature – by long years of observation, the sages discovered that particular times of the day were governed by different energies, the doshas. So it makes sense to work with, rather than against, this doshic clock.

Basically each dosha holds sway for two periods in every twenty-four hour cycle. So:

From 6am to 10am is KAPHA time

From 10am to 2pm is PITTA time

From 2pm to 6pm is VATA time

From 6pm to 10pm is KAPHA time

From 10pm to 2am is PITTA time

From 2am to 6am is VATA time

Ever wondered why you can get to sleep easily if you go to bed before 10pm but stay awake if you go at 11pm? It's because you have missed out on the relaxing, sleepy kapha time and you are becoming more stimulated thanks to the energizing pitta. Equally, have you wondered why you can eat an enormous meal at midday and not put on weight while the pounds pile on if you eat even a slightly large meal at 8pm? Fiery pitta helps midday digestion, whereas if you eat after 6pm you're into heavy kapha time. Ironically, if you're going to eat late, it's better to eat really late – after 10pm! But then you get into a whole new set of problems, so do try for that lunch-time main meal.

Just to confuse matters, ayurveda teaches that every organ has its peak time too. Morning is lung time, midday is stomach time, afternoon is liver time, and late afternoon is when the kidneys and colon rule.

All well and good, but how do you make the best use of all this knowledge? Ayurveda, as always, has the answer – a daily routine known as dinacharya.

These are its salient points.

MORNING ROUTINE

Morning is the busiest part of the ayurvedic day – this section is way longer than any of the others. At first you may think it's a physical impossibility to fit in so much before you even start your working day, but then you will notice that ayurveda advocates an early – very early – start! Don't feel you have to do it all – to begin with. It's all too easy to feel overwhelmed and then end up not doing anything. This is one reason why a lot of people are put off by ayurveda – this kind of lengthy morning routine just doesn't seem to fit with Western lifestyles. So just look on it as an ideal – maybe something you do in its entirety at weekends, or even once a month. Some parts, however, will slot quite nicely into your life – and you may be surprised to find you can do more than you think.

1   Wake up early. In an ideal ayurvedic world you would always wake up before the sun rises! That may seem like an impossibility but, if you do manage it (even once) you will notice a wonderful quality in the early morning air. There's something magical about being up while most of the (human) world around you is still slumbering. Follow the example of the birds and try getting up early – even if it's only once a week. You may soon find it addictive and

want to be an early bird all the time. But what constitutes early? Traditionally, kapha types were told to rise at a rather brisk 4.30am! Pittas were told to rise at 5.30am, while vatas had the longest lie-in – being advised to get up at a pretty civilized 6am. Try aiming for 6am to begin with and maybe slide it back a bit if you feel okay. But work with your body – don't force it. Once you start going to bed earlier (see the other end of this program!) you should find you can get up earlier.

2   Become aware. Don't race straight out of bed. Spend a few moments "coming to." Hold your hands up to your face and study them for a few moments. Become aware of your body and gently move and stretch it. Affirm to yourself that this is the start of a beautiful day and decide that you will live this day as if it were your last, fully appreciating everyone and everything you encounter. You might also want to use this quiet time to say a prayer or give thanks in some way for life.

3   Go to the bathroom. Drink a glass of water which has been allowed to stand overnight so it's at room temperature. Kapha and vata types could drink the water hot if they have sluggish bowels. This will start to stimulate your bowels. Now wash your face with cold water, splashing it gently. Clean your teeth thoroughly and also scrape your tongue. Scraping is an important part of ayurvedic routine and you can buy a special scraper from ayurvedic suppliers. Alternatively, use a spoon. Scrape gently from the back of the tongue to the front seven times so you cover the entire surface of the tongue. You should now be ready for a bowel movement so go ahead. It is a good idea to train yourself to

evacuate first thing in the morning. Even if you don't feel an urge to go, do sit on the toilet at this time every day and the habit will slowly develop.

4   Oil and bathe. Oil your entire body (see page 93 for massage techniques and oils to suit your dominant dosha). If you don't have time for a full massage, it's still worth taking time to get oil all over your skin in whatever way you can. Follow this with a bath or shower. Do it with mindfulness – paying attention to the feel of the water on your skin.

5   Take some early morning exercise. We'll discuss this more in the next chapter but for your morning regimen you will need something easy and something you can stick with! If you live near the gym, that's great. Otherwise you may need to find something you can do at or near to home. Walking is ideal and will suit all types. Jogging and running are fine if your joints can take it! Swimming is fantastic, if you have access to a pool (or, even better, the sea or an inland lake, pond or river – there's nothing quite like bathing in the natural form of the watery element, but do follow safety guidelines). Other options might include using a static bike or stepper or rower. Or investigate rebounding – aerobic exercise using a small trampoline – which is superb for mobilizing the lymphatic system as well as giving your whole body a wake-up call. Best of all for morning exercise is some yoga. The Sun Salutation (pages 69–72) was designed to send a lightning flash of energy through the entire body and to awaken the mind so it's perfect at this time. Follow it with more postures if you have time.

6 Breathe and meditate. Having done some exercise, you should sit and do some breathing or pranayama (see pages 60–65 for full details of this essential part of ayurveda). Move straight from pranayama into a period of meditation or mindfulness (see pages 84–88).

7 Breakfast. Yes, only now can you have your breakfast! And, if you are a kapha you might even be better off missing it altogether! Ideally, kapha people should have breakfast at 7am and it should be light and easily digested. Kapha can easily skip breakfast if they prefer. Pitta people should eat breakfast and should aim for 7.30am. Vata people must always eat a good breakfast and should have it at 8am.

8 Should you find you have time to spare (!!) then in an ideal ayurvedic world you would now go for a gentle fifteen to thirty minute walk. Most of us, however, will be off to work, or getting the children ready for school!

LUNCHTIME ROUTINE

1 Again, the ideal lunch time will depend on your predominant dosha. Vata should aim for early lunch between 11am and noon. Pitta should eat at high noon. Kapha can eat at the more usual time of noon to 1pm.

2 Don't race up after eating. Sit quietly for ten minutes.

3 Try, if possible, to go for a gentle walk after your lunch to aid digestion – even five minutes will help. Be mindful as you walk, aware of each step.

MID-AFTERNOON ROUTINE

If it's possible, try to find a quiet few minutes to sit and meditate or practice mindfulness. Even just two minutes will help to balance and center you.

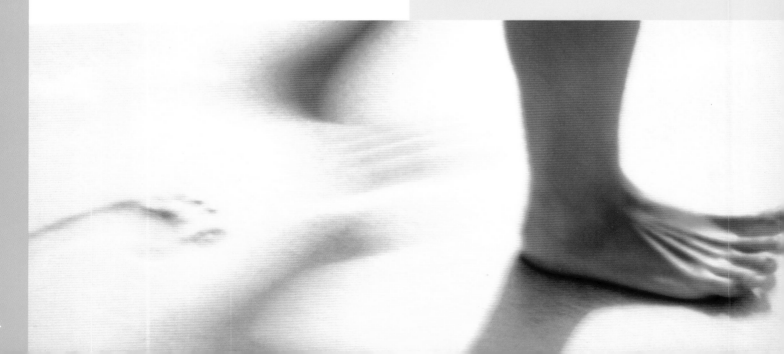

EVENING ROUTINE

1 Ideally the evening meal should be eaten around 6pm – a tough call in modern society. The traditionalists say that vata should eat at 6pm, pitta between 6pm and 7pm, while kapha can eat later at between 7pm and 8pm. Just do what you can, being aware that the earlier you eat, the better for your digestion. If you have a weight problem, then you should really aim for an early meal. Eat with awareness and don't be tempted to slump in front of the television with your supper on a tray.

2 Again, sit quietly for five minutes after you have eaten. Maybe spend this time giving thanks for the food you have eaten and thinking back over your day calmly.

3 Maybe try a gentle walk after supper. Become aware of the world winding down, the energy dipping towards sunset.

4 You may like to perform the Salutation to the Moon (see pages 76–81) as a gentle farewell to the day.

5 If you've spent the evening in lively company or watching stimulating television, spend at least a few minutes winding down and focusing on something more spiritual – reading or contemplating a mandala. Alternatively, sit quietly out in the open and listen to the sounds of nature as it shifts from day to night-time.

6 Have a milky drink. It is soothing and will help you sleep well. You may like to add some crushed almonds, which are equally soothing.

7 Rub a little sesame oil on the soles of your feet and on the top of your head (if you have time to wash your hair the next morning!) This is wonderfully soothing to the mind and prepares you for sleep.

8 Spend some time before you go to sleep in meditation. Even if you can't meditate, just sit quietly and calmly.

9 Vatas should go to bed earliest – around 10pm ideally. Pittas should follow between 10pm and 11pm. Kaphas can tolerate later nights – from 11pm to midnight.

MORAL DUTIES

Ayurveda goes beyond these practical pieces of advice. It also insists that if we want to be healthy and happy, we need to follow guidelines for our psychological health. This means that, every day, we should aim to do the following:

- Always respect those with greater wisdom than ourselves, whether they are teachers, elderly people, saints, or God. Whether you believe in God or not, or whether you meet many saints in your day-to-day life, it may be useful to consider that there will always be people and quite possibly other spiritual forces which have far greater wisdom and knowledge than ourselves. Whilst not putting ourselves down, this form of thought allows a vital sense of humility which will make us far more pleasant people to be around!

- Always try to help those who are experiencing difficulties or hardship. Kindness and generosity of spirit are called for here – and the ability to look out for others as well as ourselves. How long does it take, truly, to offer assistance to someone having difficulty crossing the road, or someone grappling to get out of a wheelchair into a car? Helping someone with heavy shopping or giving up your seat on a train to a harassed mother with a batch of kids isn't exactly difficult. Likewise, always be open to giving to charitable causes – not just offering your money but also maybe your time or expertise. A lawyer friend of mine regularly does pro bono work; another drives a bus taking disabled children on outings.

- Develop your character: be fearless, intelligent, brave, forgiving, and decisive. Phew! All pretty tough – but try every day to advance yourself in all these areas. Push yourself that bit further by doing something you would normally shy away from: hold out the hand of friendship to someone you dislike; don't allow yourself to dither; boost your intelligence by reading the broadsheets rather than the tabloids, a classic novel rather than a potboiler...

- Avoid fools, sinners, and those of a greedy nature. Ah, but sinners can be such fun! In your heart of hearts, you know the people who are good (for your soul) to be with and those who aren't. Be discriminating.

- Avoid excessive alcohol intake, drugs, and undesirable places. The ayurvedic physicians seem pretty puritanical but, in reality, it makes sense. Alcohol isn't forbidden – just over-indulgence in it, which will make you feel lousy and be bad for your health. Drugs are bad for you – it goes without saying. Undesirable places? Well, let's leave that to your conscience! But seriously, ayurveda teaches that errors of judgement can cause stress which in turn will lead to ill-health.

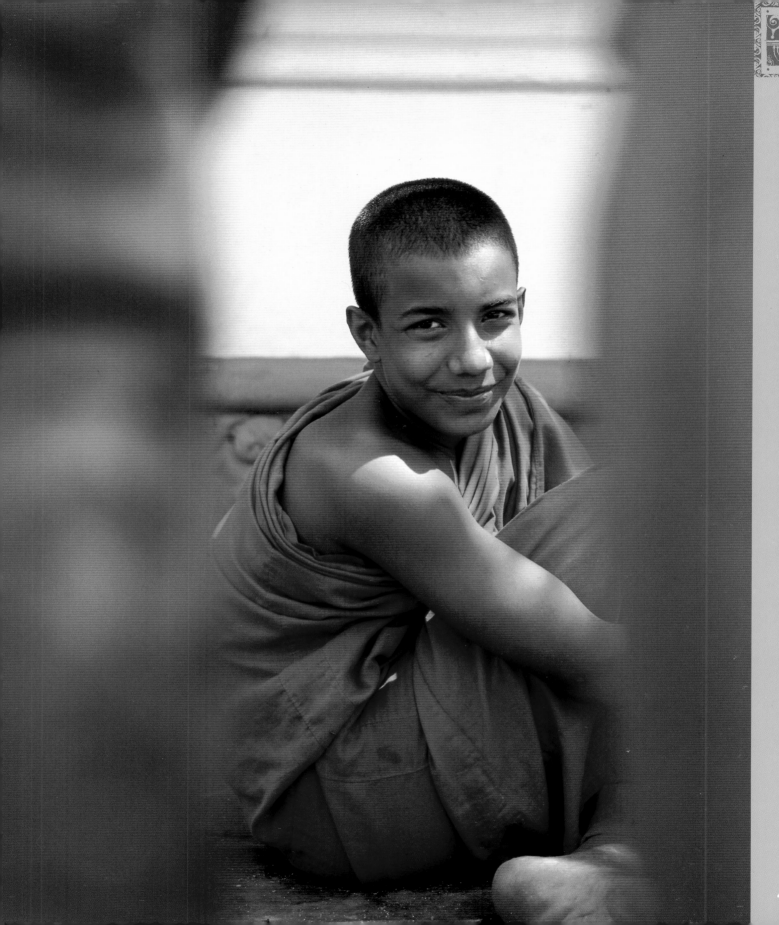

CHAPTER SIX

ideal exercise

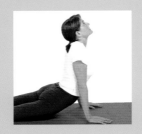

Exercise is a dirty word to many people. How many of us have tried joining the gym or going to exercise classes only to fall by the wayside after just a week or so? It can be so demoralizing that many of us simply give up altogether, which is deeply unfortunate for our health. The great news is that it's not your fault – you're probably doing the wrong form of exercise! Ayurveda can help you find the perfect exercise – one you will enjoy (honestly) and which will give you tangible results.

I hate to say this but we aren't supposed to be couch potatoes. Nature just didn't intend for us to sit for ten hours a day behind a computer screen and then slump for the rest of the evening in front of a television before falling into bed. One day we might evolve to be able to deal with our new sedentary lifestyles but, as it stands, our bodies are designed to move, to work, to be fit and active. In the past, most of us would have relied on the earth for our livelihood and our daily bread – we would have spent our days slogging pretty hard in the open air. Nowadays, our daily bread tends to come from the supermarket and so we need to find other, more artificial, ways to keep active and fit.

Do you really need to exercise? Yes, I'm afraid you do. If you want to live longer and more healthily, the single most important thing you can do (alongside a good diet) is to incorporate regular exercise into your life. Ayurveda has always taught this and modern science agrees. Exercising regularly reduces your risk of early death by an impressive 70 per cent. It keeps your lungs and heart working at optimum levels and prevents the dangers of heart disease. Stress levels drop when you exercise and your mood naturally elevates. Regular exercise can even help you sleep and perk up your sex life! On a more prosaic note, it can control your blood pressure and boost your immune system.

Some physiologists even reckon it can increase your creativity. On the other hand, if you don't exercise you are asking for trouble – you will be putting yourself in danger of heart and artery disease, your muscles and bones could develop problems, you could find yourself prone to gastrointestinal problems, and you will be more likely to suffer nervous or emotional upsets and illnesses.

The good news is that you don't have to live down the gym or run for hours every day – in fact, too *much* exercise can be bad for you as well. But you do need to do some form of exercise regularly.

So why do so many of us find exercise so darn tough? The main problem is that people take up forms of exercise they don't enjoy, they aren't naturally good at, or that they feel they *should* do. It's hardly surprising then that they get bored and disillusioned, and soon give up. Ten to one they're trying to fit themselves into the wrong activity – the proverbial square peg in the round hole.

Your ayurvedic type is the key to successful exercise. If you're a slim, slight vata you're going to be a fish out of water throwing the javelin. Conversely, a kapha isn't going to feel comfortable in a ballet class. And competitive pittas are generally going to be miserable plodding round a track on their own.

USE THE WISDOM OF AYURVEDA TO PICK YOUR IDEAL SPORT

John Douillard, a former professional athlete and ayurvedic expert, has researched the whole question of ayurveda and sport in great depth. If you want to go into this in detail I'd thoroughly recommend his excellent book *Body, Mind and Sport* (see page 202).

First and foremost, Douillard insists, fitness must be fun. The key, apparently, is to get back to the mindset we had as children, when sport and exercise was above all a game. He's quite right – as a kid I used to climb mountains for the sheer hell of it; now I find myself thinking more about how many calories I'm burning. On a recent holiday, I staggered up a peak almost chanting "100 calories, 200 calories…" and barely noticed the scenery.

Find something you actually enjoy – not what you feel you *should* do but what you would really like to do. You don't have to race out and join a tae-bo or ashtanga yoga class just because it's trendy. And you don't have to do aerobics because all your friends do or play squash because your husband wants some practice. I know so many people who have forked out a small fortune on gym memberships only to find that they hate pumping iron and they loathe step aerobics. Before you join a club, test it out for a while – any club worth its salt will offer trial memberships for a month or so.

Start to think about exercise. Take a look at your local sports center – pick up a brochure or take a wander round and I'll bet you'll be surprised at what's on offer. Think about the sports you enjoyed in school – are there any you'd like to take up again? Netball can be brilliant fun, or volleyball or softball – particularly if you like team games (kaphas are great team players). Alternatively, get back into badminton, squash or tennis (nice and competitive for pittas). Many adults take up gymnastics again and love it (they're usually vatas); or learn something new like golf. It's worth remembering that the key issue here is fun. You don't have to be brilliant or the best – you just need to do it and enjoy it. A kapha friend of mine has become a born-again belly-dancer and adores it. She reckons she's the worst belly-dancer ever but she couldn't care less.

According to ayurveda, there are two ways of looking at the exercise equation. You can examine your body type and choose a sport that suits your prakruti or you can pick something that will balance your basic nature. Let's keep it simple to begin with. If you're trying to motivate yourself to start exercise you need to choose a sport or exercise that suits your predominant dosha. Work with your natural inclinations and it will be easier to make exercise a part of your life. Later on you can think about the balancing bit.

CHOOSING A SPORT TO SUIT YOUR TYPE

VATA – You probably already exercise, as you just can't seem to sit still. Quick, light, and agile, you are not very muscular and don't have a lot of endurance.

Natural Inclinations: You're a natural for running, sprinting, hurdling, jumping – in fact any kind of track sports except long-distance or endurance running. Gymnastics, skating, ballet dancing, and fencing are great as they require agility, poise, and grace, which you have in buckets. Anything involving short bursts of energy such as squash, tennis, or badminton will be good for you. Swimming (again, usually for short lengths) and diving are great too.

PITTA – Pitta types are natural sportspeople and usually perform well in most sports as they have a combination of strength, speed, and stamina. They're also usually extremely well co-ordinated.

Natural Inclinations: The more competitive the sport the better. You'll love squash, tennis, basketball, baseball, hockey, football, rugby, and pretty well any other team or pairs sport. You'll do well at the gym with weight-training, cross-training, and circuit-training. Martial arts will appeal, as will adventurous outdoor sports such as horse-riding, rock-climbing, skiing, snowboarding, canoeing, and scuba-diving.

KAPHA – There are plenty of sports in which you will excel, as your heavier frame gives you strength and high endurance.

Natural Inclinations: Sports requiring endurance and power are your forte: any shot-putter is bound to be a kapha and most body builders have a kapha frame to build on. You do well with team sports and thrive under the motivation of others – baseball, basketball, cricket, football, and rugby are good for you. So too are volleyball and hockey. Cycling and, in particular, mountain biking, is great. Martial arts come naturally, so too does sailing, skiing (particularly cross-country), horse-riding, and golf.

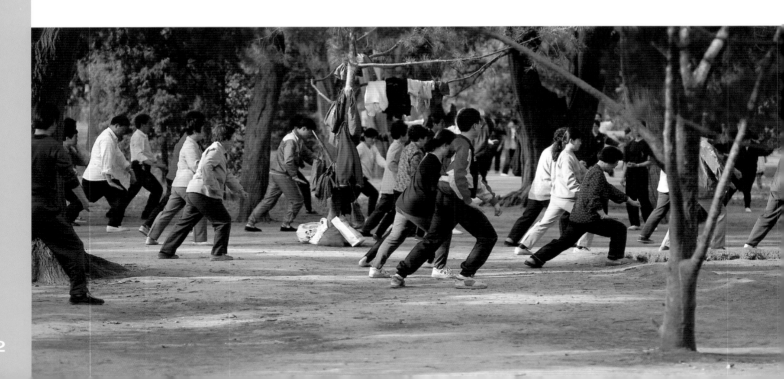

KEEPING MOTIVATION HIGH

In order to keep exercising you have to keep your motivation high. There are several key points worth remembering here:

- Be realistic about your size and body shape. Hoards of exercisers lose heart because however hard they work they don't end up looking like a supermodel or a Hollywood actress. Dump unrealistic role models – these people spend hours, and a small fortune in personal trainer bills, to look that way. If you're a kapha, you're never going to have the skinny frame of a vata – but you can be a firm, toned, beautifully strong kapha.

- Start slowly. You shouldn't try to change your exercise habits overnight or you will become demotivated because you don't see changes happening immediately. Make gradual changes to your lifestyle and they will become a permanent way of life without any special effort. Yes, that's hard for vatas in particular – but trust me and do it this way.

- Break through the one week barrier. Sports psychologists promise that if you can get past the first week, you've passed the period in which half the dropouts occur. If you manage to work out regularly for six months, you're likely to have created a longlasting habit.

- Try to get a friend involved. Exercising with someone else is the supreme motivator. Sportsmen and women have coaches, most super-fit actresses and models have their own personal trainers and if you've got the funds, a personal trainer will undoubtedly get you moving.

However, a good friend will often do as well. It is much easier to stick to a regular exercise schedule if you know that someone else is waiting for you in the park, the gym, or the pool. Choose someone around your own ability and make a commitment to your health and each other – then stick to it.

WORK WITH YOUR RHYTHMS

Many people drop out of fitness programs because they push themselves too hard at the wrong time. The key to successful, long-term fitness is to find your personal rhythms and exercise within them. Keep a notepad or calendar handy and every morning and night jot down four or five words to describe your energy level, your frame of mind, your physical condition, and what you have done workwise. After a period of time you can review and identify patterns – when certain parts of your body are tired, when exercise makes you feel great, when you're tired, when you're raring to go. Then make adjustments.

Also remember that it is not written in stone that your workout should stay exactly the same, month in, month out. Most good gyms and clubs will alter your program every few months to keep you interested and will test your fitness levels and assess your progress to keep you motivated. Cross-training will also stop you from getting bored and demoralized and has the added advantage of exercising different parts of the body and toning different muscle groups. If you always do weight-training, try a class for a change. If you have a solid routine of step and low-impact aerobics, try something different like circuit-training or Boxercise. Balance high-intensity workouts with quieter, more precise forms of exercise like yoga or chi kung.

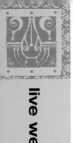

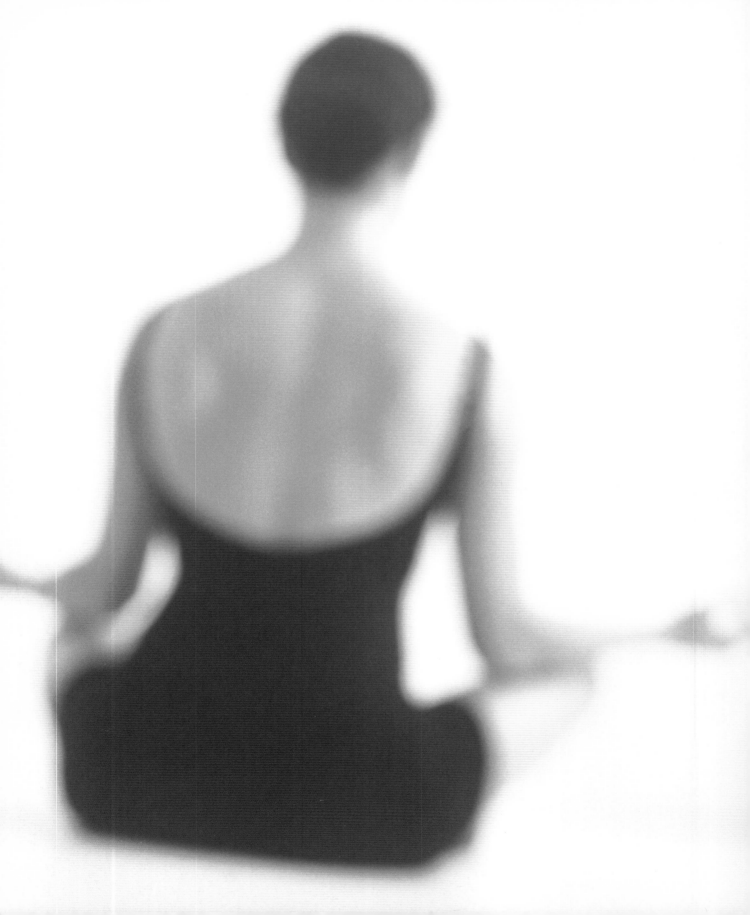

But above all, remember that exercise (in whatever form) will make a huge difference to how you look and feel. After about six weeks of regular exercise you'll notice tangible differences. Your mind should be clearer and your moods should be more balanced. Your muscles will start to feel toned. Your aerobic fitness will steadily improve and you won't be gasping if you have to walk up an escalator or run for a bus. It doesn't happen overnight but it can happen quite quickly. Once you start to notice and enjoy the benefits you'll be hooked. Why live life half-heartedly when you can enjoy it all?

BALANCING YOUR PRAKRUTI WITH SPORT

Once you're a regular exerciser and feel ready for the next step, you can use your knowledge of ayurveda to help balance your doshas. If you feel that your predominant dosha is out of balance, you can help soothe it by working out with a different form of exercise. Here's how...

VATA – If you're feeling jumpy and tense, you should try something which will soothe and calm your restless nature. Low-impact jogging or aerobics will still suit your nature but will tone down the intensity a bit. Make sure you resist the impulse to sprint or pump up the impact! Even more calming and soothing for you would be walking, hiking, cycling (gently), and swimming (again, nice and slow and rhythmic) – or how about trying synchronized swimming?

PITTA – This will be tough for you but, if you're feeling hot and bothered, tense and irritable, you need something to cool your fiery nature. In other words, anything that isn't intensely competitive. Take yourself out into nature for a spot of mountain biking, go on a long meandering hike, go swimming for the pleasure of it (resist the impulse to notch up another length or time your laps!), go cross-country skiing with a pair of binoculars to watch the wildlife, or try a leisurely round of golf (not worrying too much about your handicap).

KAPHA – If you're feeling sluggish and a bit depressed, you need speeding up and enlivening. Try out some fast sports that require endurance: squash or tennis will slough off the cobwebs. Get running or jogging – you would be a natural for a marathon if you got into shape! Rowing will work with your strengths but also provide some stimulation – and get you out into the air. Forego the gym for once and try out an aerobics class – okay, you may be a bit unco-ordinated but who cares, ignore the vatas and pittas leaping all over the place and do your own thing.

Of course, yoga works wondrously for all the types – it is soothing to all the doshas and will also help you keep flexible and fit. Try, if you possibly can, to incorporate yoga into your exercise plan. Use yoga for your stretch routine, before and after your workout. And try to do the Sun Salutation every day (see pages 69–72).

3

mind power

CHAPTER SEVEN

breathing

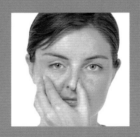

There is one ayurvedic technique which absolutely everyone should learn: breathing. Yes, we all breathe but ayurveda has elevated breathing to the status of both a science and an art form. Specific breathing techniques can help you keep your cool in difficult situations, kickstart your detox system, and send a surge of vital energy right through your entire body. In this chapter we will look at some incredibly simple techniques which will have a huge impact on your life if you make the very little effort required to practice them.

A keystone to ayurvedic health is pranayama, the art of good breathing. Breathing? Who needs to learn to breathe? You might think we're all experts in breathing: after all we've been breathing since birth, haven't we? Well that's true but there's breathing and breathing. It's a bit like saying we can all run – but compare the difference between an out-of-condition ordinary soul with an Olympic athlete. The trouble is that we take breathing for granted. We all know how to do it and so we tend to forget about it. However, if you truly want to improve your health there are few things that are more important than learning how to breathe well.

Even if you do nothing else towards helping your health on the ayurvedic path, even if you ignore every other part of this book, simply taking the trouble to learn how to breathe in the optimum way can have quite amazing benefits for you – body, mind, and spirit.

A bold claim but it's true. Breathing is our means of pulling in oxygen and circulating it around the body to "feed" each and every cell; it is also the way we send out carbon dioxide and waste products, "cleaning out" each and every cell. The better you breathe, the more effectively you nourish and clear out your body – it's as simple as that. Experts in pranayama (the technical term for the ayurvedic art and science of good breathing) say that breathing fully can do everything from improving your moods, increasing your resistance to colds and illness, fostering better sleep, and even helping you resist aging. It feeds the brain, calms the nerves, and has a measurable effect on a number of medical conditions, lowering heart rate and metabolic rate; normalizing blood pressure and decreasing the risks of cardiovascular disease.

The fundamental problem most of us have is that we breathe too shallowly, almost cautiously, only using a tiny portion of our lungs. It has been estimated that when we inhale we only take in around a tumblerful of air when we could, in fact, take in at least three times that amount. The lungs are made up of around 700 million air sacs, of which the greater proportion lie in the lower lungs. When we breathe shallowly, we don't ever quite expel all the waste gases and detritus in the lower lungs. We also run the risk of losing vital elasticity in the lower part of our lungs.

Fortunately there are very simple exercises which can help bring our breathing back to its optimum fullness and freedom. Pranayama sounds complicated but it really isn't – once you get started you'll find it's very simple and also curiously addictive. When you notice just how much difference you can make to how you feel in your body and how you can change your mood in an instant, you too will be hooked on better breathing.

Some people say that how you breathe is a good indication of how you look at life altogether. Symbolically, breathing is all about taking in the new and eliminating the old. So taking in deep joyful breaths is seen as a way of affirming life and vitality. Breathing minimally and shallowly is, in a way, turning your back on life or accepting it only grudgingly. There is a yoga proverb which says: "Life is in the breath. Therefore he who only half breathes, half lives." Who wants to half live?

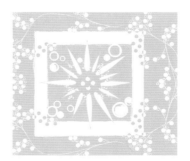

SIMPLE TECHNIQUES FOR BETTER BREATHING

Try to fit in some time each day (or weekend) to practice better breathing. But do try to do it regularly. Once you have the hang of these forms of breath you can use moments such as waiting in line, or computer breaks (yes you should have them!) to slot in a few minutes of pranayama.

THE COMPLETE BREATH

This is the basic breathing technique of pranayama. It is an excellent training tool as it encourages you to breathe fully, bringing oxygen deep into the cells and pulling out toxins. It is also incredibly calming. If you ever find yourself in a situation when you need to be relaxed, just bring your breathing into this pattern – you will immediately find your heart-rate decelerate and your mind begin to clear. You will learn how to do this breath lying on the floor, as this makes it easy to feel what's happening. Once you're expert in it you will be able to do it anywhere. You will find this form of breathing a very handy tool when we come to learn how to meditate later on in this section of the book.

1 Lie down on the floor and make yourself comfortable. Bring your feet close in to your buttocks and allow the feet to fall apart, bringing the soles of the feet together, hands resting gently on your abdomen with the fingertips gently touching. This posture stretches the lower abdomen, which enhances the breathing process.

2 Breathe in with a slow, smooth inhalation through your nostrils, feeling your abdomen expand. Your fingers will part as your abdomen expands.

3 Exhale slowly and steadily through your nostrils, noticing that your abdomen flattens and that your fingers are once again touching.

4 Pause for a second or two and then repeat this inhalation and exhalation, becoming conscious of the movement of the breath down through your chest and abdomen. Breathe at your own pace in this way for around five minutes or as long as you feel comfortable.

5 If you feel comfortable with this you can extend the breath into the chest. Once the inhalation has filled the abdomen simply continue to inhale, feeling the chest expand. This provides a longer, deeper breath.

6 Finally, bring your knees together and gently stretch out the legs. Allow yourself to relax comfortably on the ground for a few minutes (place a cushion under your lower back or your neck if you wish).

ALTERNATE NOSTRIL BREATHING

This classic pranayama technique feels rather strange to begin with but, once you become used to it, is very soothing. It is particularly useful if you are feeling stressed or anxious or if you cannot sleep at night.

1   Sit comfortably in a chair, with both feet on the floor. Don't slouch. Gently allow your eyes to close, your body to relax, and your mind to still.

2   Place your dominant hand around your nose. If you are right-handed, the most natural way to do this will be to place your right thumb against your right nostril with the rest of the fingers of your right hand lying gently across your left nostril. The aim is to close off one nostril at a time, comfortably and easily, without constantly moving your hand.

3   Pressing with the thumb, gently close the right nostril and slowly exhale through your left nostril. Note that you are starting the breath on an exhale. Now inhale through the same nostril.

4   Next close off the left nostril, exhale through the right, and inhale again. Allow your breath to be smooth and relaxed. Don't try to breathe very deeply – keep it natural. You may find you need to blow your nose a lot – don't worry, that's perfectly normal.

5   Alternate between the two nostrils for around five minutes if you can. If you feel uncomfortable at any time, breathe through your mouth for a while until you can go back to the nose.

6   When you've finished, allow yourself to simply sit and relax with your eyes closed for a while.

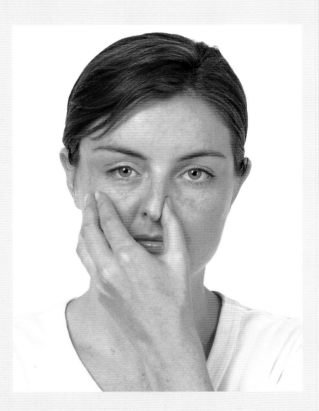

DETOX BREATH

This is a superb breathing exercise that improves elimination of toxins from the body. It strengthens the lungs, massages and tones the abdominal muscles, and refreshes the nervous system. However, do not practice it if you have a heart condition, high blood pressure, epilepsy, hernia, or any ear, nose, or eye problems. Also avoid it if you are pregnant or menstruating (see Note below.)

1   Choose your position. This exercise can be performed sitting, standing, or lying down. Whichever you choose, make sure you are comfortable and relaxed. Breathe regularly and normally.

2   Inhale slowly, smoothly, and deeply but do not strain your breathing.

3   Now exhale briskly, as if you were sneezing. Focus your attention on your abdomen – it will automatically flatten and tighten as you exhale.

4   Allow yourself to inhale naturally – it will happen automatically following the brisk exhale.

5   Now continue breathing in this way for a few minutes – or as long as you feel comfortable. It is a brisk technique and very energetic so don't be surprised if you only manage a minute or so to begin with.

6   Resume normal breathing and relax.

Note – If you are pregnant or menstruating you can use a modified form of this exercise. Instead of the "sneezing" exhale, pout your lips and allow your breath to come out through in a steady stream, as if you were blowing out candles on a cake. This is a much slower technique than the basic detox breath and excellent if you need to calm down in a difficult situation.

CHAPTER EIGHT

yoga – stretch to fresh limits

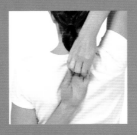

Yoga is incredibly fashionable at the moment and there are various kinds of classes available virtually everywhere. Yoga is much more than just a trendy fad though: it's a superlative system which will stretch your muscles and your mind. A yoga workout is the perfect form of exercise for all ages, shapes, and temperaments, and is also very clever: at the end of a session you should feel both wildly energized and yet superbly calm. If you're still not tempted, just remember that regular yoga practice not only makes you feel better but will without question make you look better too.

Yoga is deceptive. You watch someone in a yoga posture (called an asana) and it looks so simple you think it can't possibly be having much effect. But rest assured it is. Like all of ayurveda, hatha yoga (the physical form of yoga) has been perfected over many thousands of years – every posture is specifically designed to have a precise physiological, psychological, and spiritual effect on your body and mind.

On a purely physical level, yoga puts pressure on all the different organs and muscles of the body very systematically. As well as toning the outer body, it tones the whole inner body: the liver, the lungs, the kidneys, the spleen, the intestines, the heart. Yoga practitioners say that the precise asanas of yoga work deep into the body, causing blood to circulate profoundly rather than just around the outside edge of the body, nourishing every organ and softening the muscle and ligament tissue. The deep stretching is said to bring both bones and muscles gently back into their optimum alignment while lubricating the joints.

Yoga can improve the oxygenation of your blood and improve your circulation. It's also a superb way of helping your body to detox, as it encourages the discharge of toxins. Not only does your body detox while you perform yoga; your mind does too. The breathing directly affects the nervous system, eliciting the "relaxation response" in which the parasympathetic nervous system takes over from the sympathetic nervous system so you feel calm, cool, and in control.

Hopefully you will already be doing the stretching exercises you learned at the start of this book. These will stand you in good stead as you begin yoga. If not, don't worry – you can perform these postures without any prior knowledge, but do take it easy to begin with.

Caution

Just like any form of exercise, yoga can harm as well as heal if practiced incorrectly. Note the following:

- Don't push yourself beyond your limits. Yoga is not competitive (pittas please note!) – everyone works at their own pace and within their body's limits. It's tempting to over-stretch but start very gently – you will soon find you can stretch further.

- If you have any health problems (particularly heart conditions, back problems, or if you have had any kind of surgery) you should find a yoga therapist (who has had a strict medical training) rather than a yoga teacher.

- If you are pregnant, you will need to avoid certain postures. Again, you should see a yoga therapist or find a class specifically designed for pregnant women.

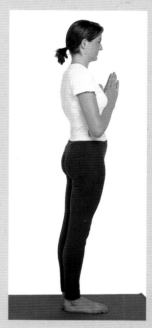

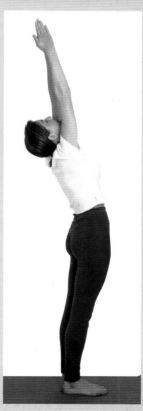

THE SUN SALUTATION

A COMPLETE WORKOUT FOR BODY, MIND, AND SPIRIT

The Sun Salutation or Salute to the Sun is a popular yoga routine. It is becoming well-known (and deservedly so) because it is perhaps the most effective series of exercises you can do for your body. It systematically stretches virtually every muscle in your body and massages the internal organs as well. In ancient India it was part of daily spiritual practice and was performed in the very early morning facing the sun, the deity for health and long life. If you can, try to practice this simple series of poses every day – if you can do it first thing in the morning, so much the better. If you can do it at dawn and really greet the sun, you are a better person than I and you'll undoubtedly reap the benefits.

If you do just this one exercise on a daily basis you will become far more flexible, particularly in your spine. You will also increase your breathing capacity and help the elimination of toxins. It can even help reduce a fat tummy. The series of exercises involves twelve spinal positions and each stretches different ligaments and moves the spine in different ways. At first the transition from one posture to the next will seem jerky and uncoordinated, but do persevere. As you begin to learn them off by heart you will find you can move fluidly and smoothly from one to another. Start off by doing just one whole set and gradually build up to the optimum twelve (some ayurvedic sages say you should perform one set of the salutation for every year of your life!) You may find it helpful to record the instructions on a tape recorder until you become familiar with them.

1   Standing upright, bring your feet together so your big toes are touching. Your arms are by your sides. Relax your shoulders and tuck your chin in slightly – look straight ahead, not down at your feet. Bring your hands together in front of your chest with palms together as if you were praying. Exhale deeply.

2   Inhale slowly and deeply while you bring your arms straight up over your head, placing your palms together as you finish inhaling. Gently tilt your head backwards and look towards your thumbs. Lift the knee caps by tightening your thighs. Reach up as far as possible, lengthening your whole body. If you feel comfortable you can take the posture back slightly further into a bend.

3 Exhale as you bend forwards and place your hands on the floor in line with your feet. Try to get your head as close to your knees as possible. To begin with you might find you have to bend your knees in order to get close. Eventually you should be able to straighten your knees into the full posture.

4 Inhale deeply and move your right leg away from your body in a big backwards sweep so you end up in a kind of extended lunge position. Keep your hands and left foot firmly on the ground. Your left knee should be between your hands. Bend your head upwards, stretching out your back.

5 Take your left leg back and, exhaling deeply, bring yourself into an arched position. Your arms are in front of your head, palms facing directly in front, arms shoulder-width apart. Your back should be in a straight line with your head in line with your arms. Keep your feet and heels flat on the floor. This posture is known as the Dog.

6 Exhale and lower your body onto the floor. Only eight parts of your body should be in contact with the floor: your feet, your knees, your hands, your chest, and your forehead. Try to keep your abdomen raised and, if you can possibly manage it, keep your nose off the floor so only your forehead makes contact. Don't worry if it's an impossibility at this point – just keep the idea in mind.

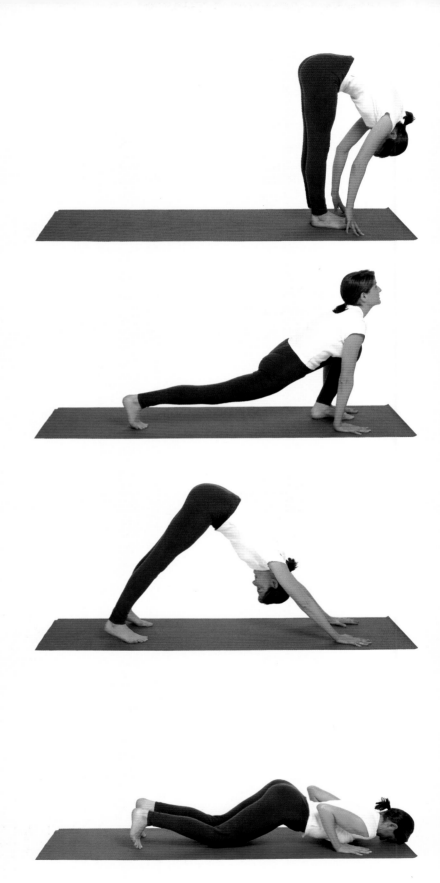

7 Inhale and bend up into the position known as the Cobra – with your hands on the floor in front of you, arms straight, bend backwards as far as feels comfortable. Look upwards.

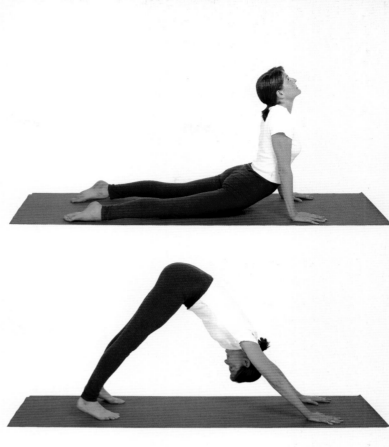

8 Exhale and lift your back to return to the position in step 5. Remember to keep your feet and heels flat on the floor if you can.

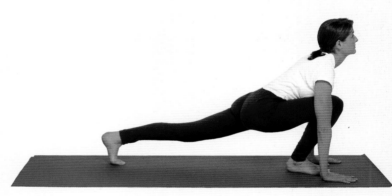

9 Inhale and return to the step 4 position, this time with the opposite leg forwards. Your right foot should be in line with your hands while your left leg is stretched back.

10 Exhale and return to step 3.

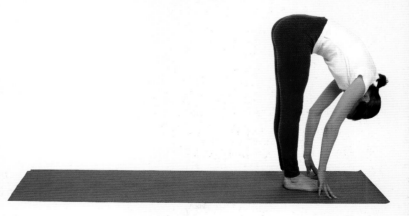

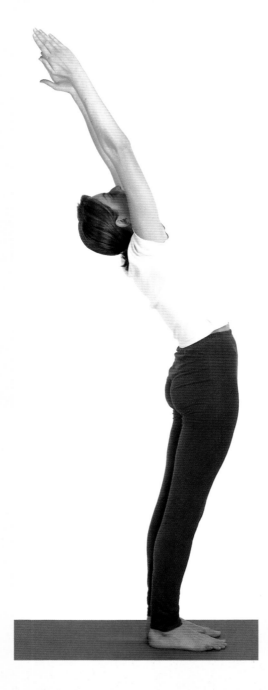

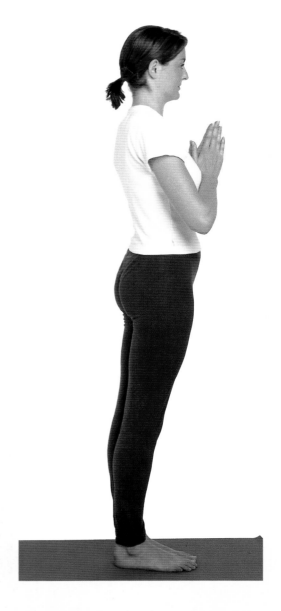

11 Raise the arms overhead and bend backwards as you inhale (as for step 2).

12 Return to a comfortable standing position, feet together, arms by your sides. Look straight ahead and exhale. To finish, bring your hands back together in a position of prayer.

FURTHER YOGA POSTURES FOR HEALTH AND VITALITY

As you become more proficient in yoga, you can extend your practice. Once you have performed your sun salutations, you may like to include the following postures, all of which will help to increase your vital energy, clear your mind, and purify your body. Perform them slowly and carefully in a controlled manner. Never rush. It's better to do just one posture carefully and thoughtfully than the whole bunch half-heartedly and in a slipshod manner.

THE MOUNTAIN

This seated variation of the mountain posture tones your abdominal muscles and improves your breathing. It can help sluggish circulation and can also tone the muscles in the back.

1   Sit cross-legged on the floor. Hold yourself upright and breathe naturally and easily.

2   Inhale and stretch your arms up over your head to form a steeple shape over your head. Keep the insides of your arms close to your ears. Bring your palms together if you can and press them together as if you were praying.

3   Hold this posture for as long as you comfortably can. Remember to breathe easily and regularly as you hold the pose.

4   Exhale and slowly lower your arms to your lap. Rest for a few moments and then repeat.

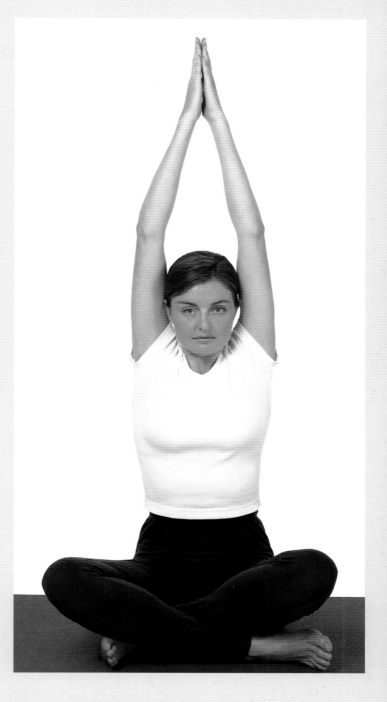

PRAYER POSTURE

This gentle posture puts all your internal organs into balance. It encourages deep breathing and helps to align your spine into its optimum position. It is also deeply calming for the mind.

1 Stand with your feet together and parallel. Aim to stand tall without straining – imagine you have a string fastening your head to the ceiling.

2 Check your head – it should be easily balanced on your neck with eyes gazing softly ahead. Your chin should be neither tucked in nor jutting out.

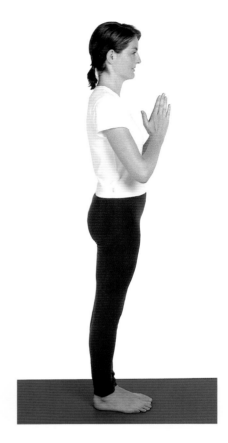

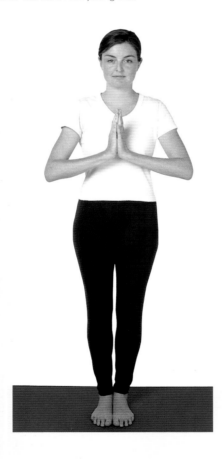

3 Tilt your pelvis slightly forwards and keep your knees straight but soft – don't lock them.

4 Now bring your hands together in front of your chest, as if you were praying.

5 Relax your jaw, your facial muscles, and your shoulders. Breathe softly and regularly. You may want to focus lightly on an object in front of you, or you can gently close your eyes.

6 Hold this pose for a few minutes or as long as you feel comfortable. Then bring your hands back down to your sides and resume your normal stance.

THE TREE

A classic yoga posture which is superb for improving balance, concentration, and coordination.

1   Stand up tall and straight. Your feet should be close together and parallel. Fix your eyes gently on a spot directly ahead of you and breathe naturally and regularly. You will need to keep your eyes open for this posture.

2   Lift one leg and place the sole of your foot against the inner side of your other thigh. You can use your hands to help. Keep focusing on the point ahead of you.

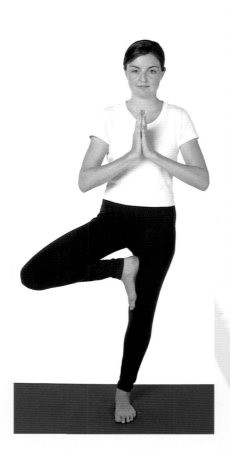

3   Now bring your hands up in a prayer position in front of your chest.

4   Hold the posture for as long as feels comfortable. Focus on your breathing and think about the strength and poise of a tree – its roots firm in the ground, its branches reaching towards heaven.

5   Repeat the posture standing on the other leg.

CHILD POSTURE

This posture may seem very simple but has very deep effects. It massages your internal organs, promoting good circulation and helping elimination. It also helps to keep your spine supple and flexible, and is excellent if you suffer from lower back pain.

1   Kneel down with your feet pointing backwards and your legs together. Lower your buttocks so you are sitting on your heels.

2   Now bend forwards slowly until your forehead is resting on the floor before you. You may not be able to get this far – don't worry, just go as far as is comfortable. If it helps, you can rest your head on a cushion.

3   Take your arms behind you so your hands rest on the floor next to your feet, palms facing upwards. Relax.

4   Stay in this posture for as long as you feel comfortable. Try to keep your breathing regular and relaxed.

SALUTATION TO THE MOON

For quite some time I thought it was a bit unfair that we can salute the sun but not the moon. Then I discovered this lovely sequence. Just as you celebrated the rise of the sun at the beginning of your day, so you can salute the cooling, calming energy of the moon at the end of the day. This series of postures, performed like the Sun Salutation, in a continuous sequence, can help balance the body and psyche for the night ahead. Start with one or two repetitions and gradually build up. Again, you may want to record the instructions.

1   Stand upright, feet shoulder-width apart, knees softly bent. Your arms are hanging loosely by your sides. Your head is balanced easily on your neck – you might imagine a string attached to the very top of your head gently pulling you up into alignment.

2   Inhale gently and raise both arms up over the head, gently bending the upper body and head back as far as you can comfortably go.

3   Exhale gently, slowly bringing the arms forward. Bend your torso forwards, keeping your legs straight, and touch the floor with your palms.

4   Inhale gently, bend the knees and lower your buttocks slowly into a squat. Exhale.

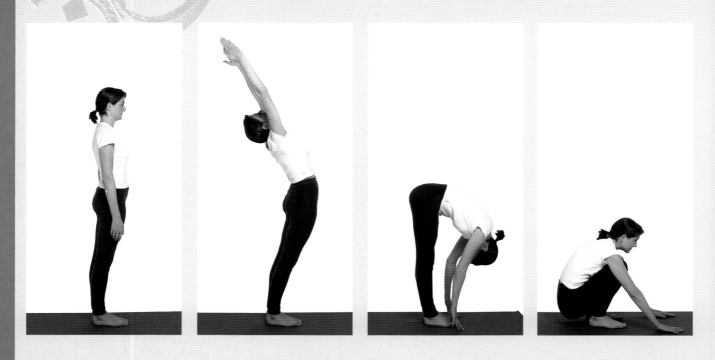

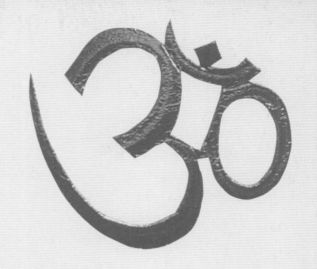

5 Inhale gently. Extend the left leg back with the knee
   touching the floor. Raise your arms over your head and
   bend your upper body back into the pose known
   as the Flag.

6 Exhale gently, bringing your palms down to the floor, and
   stretch your body forward as far as possible into the Leg
   Spread posture.

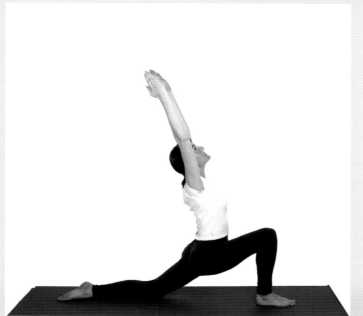

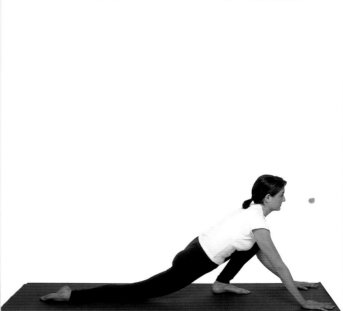

7 Inhale gently and bring your right knee back to rest on the floor beside your left knee. Standing on your knees, raise your arms up over your head and gently bend your body back as far as you can comfortably go. This is known as the Half Moon posture.

8 Exhale gently and bring your arms and torso down and forward, lowering your buttocks to rest on your calves. Touch your head on the floor and bend forwards into the Tortoise position.

9 Inhale gently and bring your torso along the floor by bending your arms and then straightening them, pushing your head, shoulders, and torso back into the Cobra position.

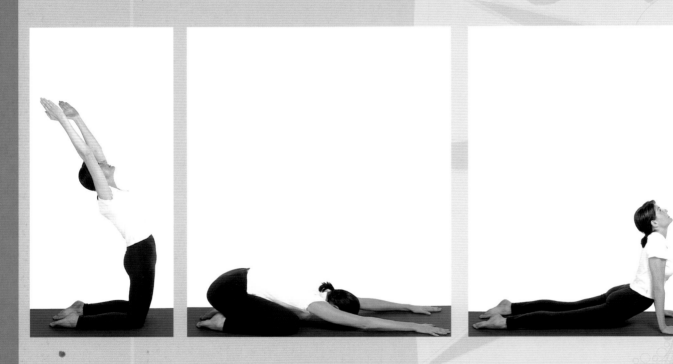

10 Exhale gently and return to step 8 – the Tortoise.

11 Inhale gently, raise yourself up on your knees and return to step 7 – the Half Moon.

12 Exhale gently, bring your palms down to the floor and return to step 6 – the Leg Spread.

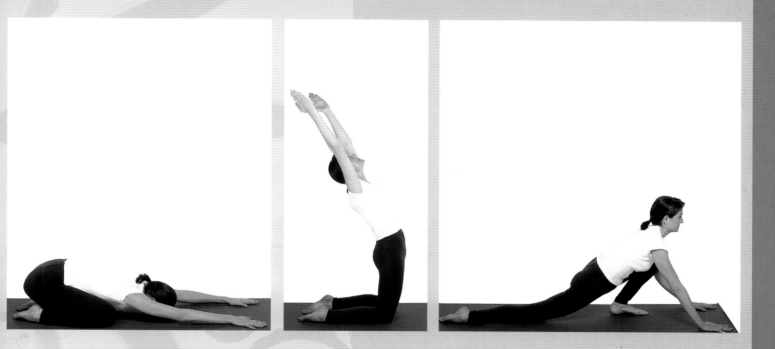

CHAPTER NINE

meditation and mindfulness

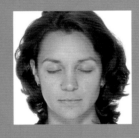

Modern day meditators fall over themselves to tell non-converts how brilliant their mind games are. They swear a daily dose of meditation makes them calmer, clearer, more able to make decisions, and way more creative. None of this is any surprise to followers of ayurveda, which has been preaching the wonders of meditation for five thousand years. Meditation need not be a chore – and it need not be difficult. There are forms of meditation to suit every soul and every time frame. If you've never tried it, give it a go. If you've tried before and failed, maybe it's time to give it a second chance.

BRINGING MINDFULNESS INTO EVERYDAY LIFE

Start each day with mindfulness. Wake up a little earlier than usual (hopefully you're already doing this as part of your daily routine) and before you even move notice your breathing; breathe consciously for a few minutes. Feel your body lying in bed and then straighten it out and stretch. Try to think of the day ahead as an adventure, filled with possibilities. Remember, you can never really know what the day will hold.

- Try stopping, sitting down, and becoming aware of your breathing once in a while throughout the day. It can be for five minutes or even five seconds. Just breathe and let go, allowing yourself to be exactly as you are.

- Set aside a time every day to just be: five minutes would be fine, or twenty or thirty. Sit and become aware of your breath and every time your mind wanders, simply return to the breath.

- Use your mindfulness time to contemplate what you really want from life. Ask yourself questions like, "Who am I?" "Where am I going?" "If I could choose a path now, in which direction would I head?" "What do I truly love?" You don't have to come up with answers, just persist in asking the question.

- Try getting down on the floor once a day and stretch your body mindfully, if only for three or four minutes. Stay in touch with your breathing and listen to what your body has to tell you.

- Use ordinary occasions to become mindful. When you are in the shower, really feel the water on the skin rather than losing yourself in thought. When you eat, really taste your food. Notice how you feel when the phone rings.

- Practice kindness to yourself. As you sit and breathe, invite a sense of self-acceptance and cherishing to arise in your heart. If it starts to go away, gently bring it back. Imagine you are being held in the arms of a loving parent, completely accepted and completely loved.

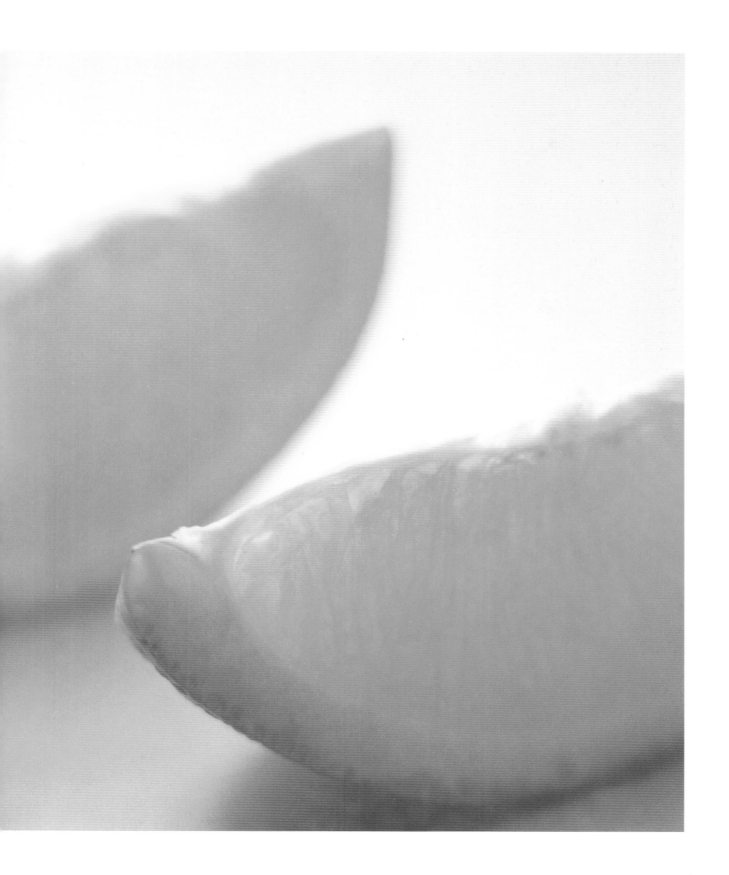

4

stimulate and soothe
your senses

massage miracles

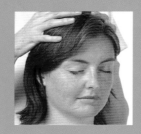

Is there anything more wonderful in life than a good massage? In a society deprived of touch, massage is nothing short of a miracle. Quite apart from its therapeutic effect on taut muscles, bodywork puts us back in touch with our bodies and our emotions. Ayurveda has had five thousand years to perfect its massage therapies and they are some of the most spectacular on the planet. If you have the chance to experience them from a professional, jump at it! For those who don't have the opportunity to enjoy such a treat, this chapter looks at some ways you can re-create the experience at home.

If so far you have found ayurveda a rough, tough ride, relax! This is the point at which it really does become a super feel-good therapy. After all, how many physicians do you know who would prescribe a massage every day! Perhaps they should take a leaf out of ayurveda's book.

Massage is finally becoming recognized as the wonder-treatment it really is. Numerous studies have shown that touch has the power to affect us on all levels. A good session of bodywork won't just affect your body but also your mind and essential well-being. First of all, the soothing touch of hands on skin stimulates the parasympathetic nervous system into a state of deep relaxation, thus making massage superlative for offsetting the ill-effects of stress. Secondly, massage builds up the body's strength and helps to build stamina. And lastly, on a cosmetic level (not to be sniffed at), it makes your skin look softer, smoother, and remarkably more youthful. Ayurvedic massage often uses oils – boosted with herbs and spices – which deeply penetrate the body: it's like giving your body an oil change and a full service!

So far we haven't even looked at the psychological effects. Virtually everyone who works with bodies – from acupuncturists to zero balancers, from reflexologists to Rolfers – is aware that we hold memories in our tissue and that when our bodies are moved those holding patterns can be released. As a result, it's not uncommon for people to relive old experiences whilst on the massage table. Other people find they don't actually remember anything in particular but have a sense that something has been lifted from them – as one massage therapist told me, "It's like having psychotherapy but without having to delve into the painful stuff: bodywork can just release old traumas without having to relive them."

THE VARIOUS FORMS OF MASSAGE

Ayurveda encompasses a host of massage techniques, so there's usually something to suit every kind of person and every kind of problem. If you visit an ayurvedic center you will most likely find the following massage therapies are used regularly. They are all classic ayurvedic massage techniques and absolutely wonderful – every body deserves to be pampered with them at least once, and by then you're hooked for life!

ABHYANGA – an incredibly relaxing massage which is designed to stimulate both the release of toxins from the cells and circulation to the subcutaneous tissues. It's an oil massage performed by two people working in perfect synchronization. There are three types of basic abhyanga, depending on your type. They vary in depth and speed of stroke, and usually take from 35 minutes to an hour. Pinda Abhyanga is similar but uses a herbalized milk and rice mixture that nourishes and feeds the skin. This massage has a wonderful effect on dry, rough skin – softening it and giving it a silky sheen.

VISHESH – a firm, squeezing massage that is designed to remove deeply-rooted toxins. It is a very strong massage, particularly suited to kapha people.

URDVARTANA – an invigorating massage using a specially blended herbalized paste made with grain, flour, herbs, and oils. It cleanses, exfoliates, tones, and tightens the skin, leaving it feeling fresh, young, and smooth. It increases circulation, promotes weight loss, and is very effective against cellulite.

GARSHAN – the use of raw silk gloves in this brisk, enlivening therapy creates friction and static electricity on the surface of the skin. It promotes weight loss and exfoliates and stimulates the skin, helping to clear away impurities.

PIZZICHILI – literally gallons of warm oil are poured over your body while two therapists gently massage in the oil. The oil deeply penetrates the skin and is especially good for releasing deep-seated aches and pains, and bringing flexibility to the joints. Pizzichili is known as the "royal treatment" as it was once the preserve of Indian royalty.

SWEDENA – this therapy softens and dilates the channels of the body, allowing impurities to move out, ready to be eliminated. After a massage, a tent is erected over the body, with the head remaining outside. The tent is then filled with a continuous flow of herbalized steam which surrounds the body, while the head is kept cool with applications of coconut oil and cool, water-soaked towels.

SHIRODHARA – a stream of oil is poured continuously over the forehead to a specific pattern and temperature. It is very effective for balancing and settling vata disorders such as insomnia, anxiety, and worry. Shirodhara is a blissful treatment which settles the mind and profoundly relaxes the central nervous system, giving the effect of a deep, silent meditative state.

NETRA TARPANA – relaxes, soothes, and relieves eyes that are aching from the effects of computers and pollution. Following a face massage, hot towels are wrapped gently around the face. Dough rings are then placed around the eyes and filled with special cooling oils to cover and bathe the eyes.

KATI BASTI – an external, localized application of massage in which heat and specific herbalized oils are used in the region of the lower back. This therapy relieves lower back pain and eases rigidity of the lower spine, strengthening the bone tissue in that area.

SHIRO BASTI – an unusual but effective therapy which is administered to the head in a special container which looks like a hat. Warm, herbalized oil is poured into the container and left for twenty minutes for the oil to be fully absorbed into the scalp. This therapy is very useful for headaches and memory loss, as well as being soothing and settling in general.

HOME MASSAGE CLASS

Obviously many of the ayurvedic massages involve highly specialized techniques which require well-trained therapists. However, several of them are quite easy to learn and can be highly effective when used at home.

The basic ayurvedic massage is a simple oil "bath" – literally dousing the entire body with oil. This is very soothing for vata and calming for pitta. It is also relaxing for kapha, but too much oil can overload the oily kapha system so kaphas need to use oil sparingly. Oiling has a huge array of benefits: it opens and cleanses the pores, increases blood circulation, reduces fat, rejuvenates the skin, calms the nerves, and soothes the psyche. Apparently it even helps strengthen bones. And, of course, it feels fantastic. Ideally, find someone to massage you – it's far more relaxing that way. Perhaps you could trade massages. If that's not feasible, it's still quite possible to achieve good results with a self-massage.

CHOOSING THE RIGHT OIL

Ayurveda specifies certain oils depending on your type.

VATA: Sesame oil is the first choice, although olive and almond oil can be used on the body. If the weather is very hot and the vata person is hot, choose coconut oil as it has a cooling effect.

PITTA: Cooling coconut oil is usually the best choice for pitta. If the weather is very cold, choose sesame oil instead.

KAPHA: Use less oil on a typical kapha person. A little sesame oil is good for kapha and mustard oil is also useful for body massage. If it's very hot and the kapha person is hot, choose a little coconut oil.

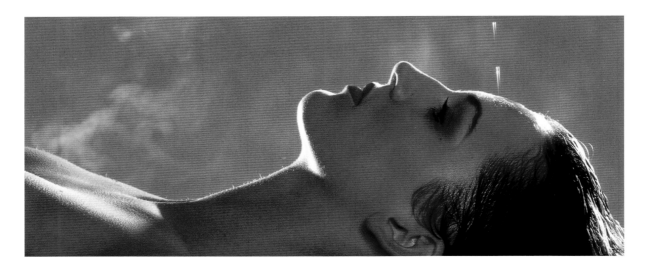

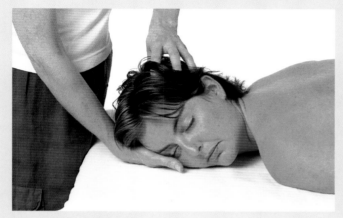

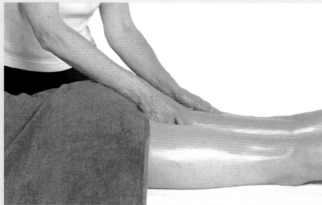

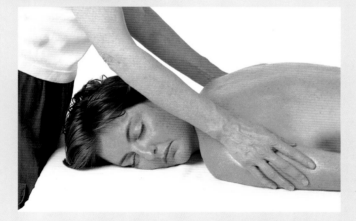

HOW TO MASSAGE

For your massage, choose a warm, comfortable room that is free from clutter and drafts. Place a large warmed towel on the floor and ask the person to lie on their front. Ideally they should be naked (oil will stain clothes) – if modesty dictates, wear (old) pants or a piece of muslin as a loin cloth. You may want to cover the parts not being massaged with towels. If you are massaging yourself, it may be easier to sit upright. Warm the chosen oil to body temperature by placing the container of oil in a bain marie of hot water.

The most usual ayurvedic massage touch is light, rhythmic, and repetitive. As a general rule of thumb, use circular movements over rounded areas such as joints and straight strokes over straight areas such as the arms, legs, and neck. There's no need to learn a whole battery of techniques – the aim is simply to introduce the oil to the body and soothe the body.

1   Start with the head. Massage the oil gently into the scalp and down the neck.

2   Continue down the back and onto the hips and buttocks. Keep your touch light and rhythmic. Work down each leg in turn and pay particular attention to the feet (these can take firmer pressure). Don't forget to massage between each toe.

3   Move back to the shoulders and work down each arm to the tips of the fingers, making sure every inch is covered with oil. Take your time – don't rush.

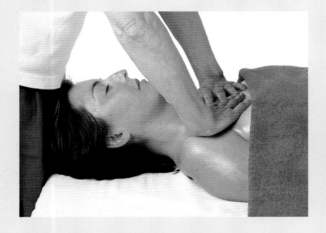

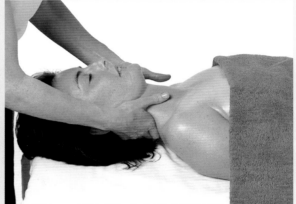

4   Quietly ask your subject to turn over. Massage the arms, legs, chest (traditional ayurvedic massage always includes massaging a woman's breasts but not everyone will feel comfortable with that, so check with your subject first), and abdomen.

5   Now move to the neck and face. Pay particular attention to every part of the face – make your movements very gentle. Work gently inside each nostril. Pull the ear lobes (give them each a firm tug) and massage gently inside the ear (but don't poke – keep your fingers on the first ridge of the ear).

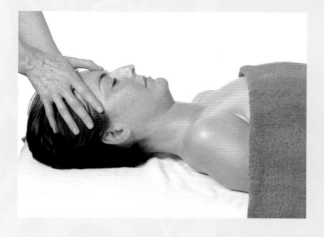

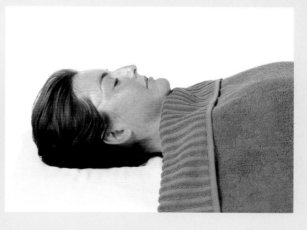

6 Finish by spending quite some time (at least five minutes) gently massaging the third eye area (just above and between the eyebrows) with your thumb.

7 Make sure your subject is warm (it's probably a good idea to cover them with old towels or blankets) and leave them to relax for between 15 and 30 minutes.

GARSHAN

Unlike many of the ayurvedic massage techniques, Garshan doesn't use oil. It is a highly stimulating treatment which boosts circulation, digestion, detoxification, and metabolism. For these reasons it is ideal if you are trying to lose weight or detox your system. Perform garshan before a bath or shower – ideally in the morning. Traditionally, garshan is performed with a pair of "gloves" made of raw silk. Raw silk is readily available from fabric shops and you can easily make a pair: spread your fingers and lay your hand on the fabric, draw loosely around it, cut out two copies, sew them together, then incorporate a piece of elastic around the wrist.

This massage is quite vigorous so use a fair amount of pressure and quite a swift action. You need to use long strokes over the large, long bones of the body and circular movements over the joints. Start by using ten strokes per area and gradually build up to around forty or fifty.

1 Start with the head, using circular movements, then stroke firmly down the neck and along the shoulder.

2 Use a circular motion over the shoulder joints then, using long strokes, sweep down the upper arms. Circle around the elbows and sweep down the forearms. Circle around the wrists and then finish up with long strokes over the hands to the tips of the fingers.

3 Now move to the chest and use long strokes across the chest, from side to side, avoiding the area directly over the heart and breasts.

4 Move down to the abdomen and stroke from side to side, then diagonally across the abdomen. Work vigorously over the hips and buttocks.

5 Now move down the legs. Use long strokes down the thighs, circling over the knees; then long strokes down the calves, circling around the ankles. Finish with long strokes down to the toes.

HEAD MASSAGE

Head massage, or champissage, is considered an important part of ayurveda. It can help cure headaches and will ease conditions such as sinusitis, colds, and migraine. It is also supposed to help improve your memory.

Use coconut, sesame, or olive oil (see page 96 for the best choice). Your massage should ideally last around 20–30 minutes. Depending on whether you use soft or vigorous movements, it will either relax or energize your partner. Before you start, make sure your hands are well-washed and your nails scrupulously clean. Ask your partner to remove glasses, contact lenses, and any jewelry. Your partner does not need to undress for the massage but, if you are using oil, they may want to wear an old, loose top or wrap up in a large towel.

The oil should be warm but not hot, so stand it on or near a radiator for around half an hour, or place it in a microwave for a minute.

Note Do not perform head massages on someone who has a skin condition such as weeping eczema or psoriasis, or if there are any open cuts or sores on their head.

1 Have your partner sit upright in a straight-backed chair. Gently lay your hands on the crown of your partner's head and just hold them there for around 30 seconds. Slowly begin to massage the scalp with the pads of your fingertips. Use just enough oil to lubricate the scalp.

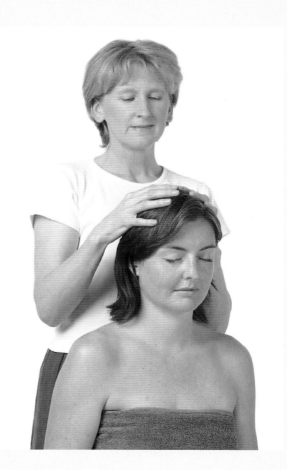

101

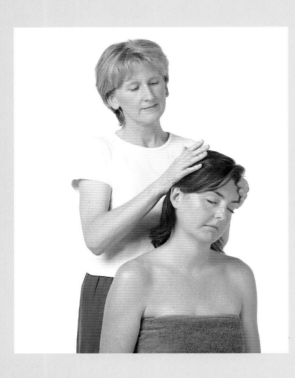

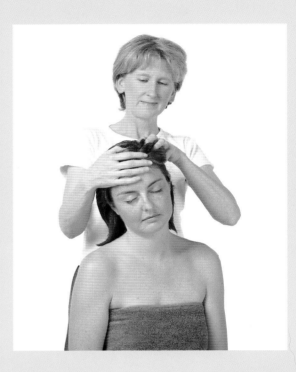

2 Now support the head with one hand. Using the palm of your other hand employ a swift rubbing motion, as if you were buffing a window. Start behind the ear, go around it, and then away from the ear. Repeat on the other side of the head. This relaxes and warms the muscles.

3 Next, support the head with one hand while the other gently strokes the top of the head. First use long sweeping movements, then "comb" the hair, running your fingernails through the hair in long strokes. Work all the way around the head, swapping hands where necessary. This stimulates blood flow through the scalp and gives a lovely tingly feeling to the head.

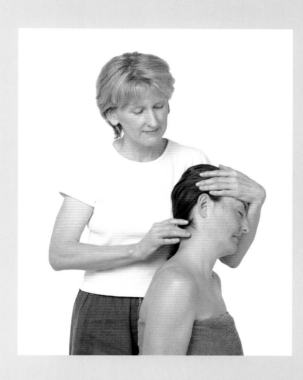

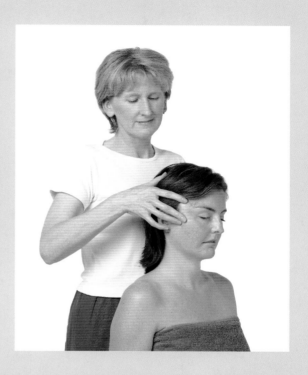

4   Take the weight of your partner's head on your arm. Now, starting at the top of the neck (where it joins the cranium), massage down either side of the spine using small circling movements of the thumb and middle finger. Go carefully and be aware of how your partner reacts – don't press too deeply. This stroke soothes and calms the brain itself.

5   Massage the temples with the tips of the index fingers, using gentle circular movements. Now support the back of the head with your hands and use a firmer (but still soft) pressure, massaging the temples with your thumbs.

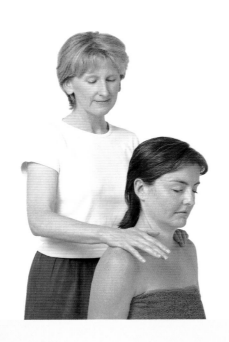

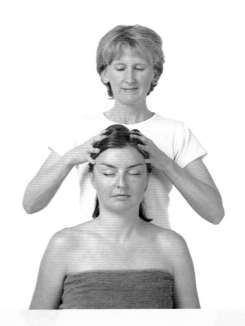

6 Now concentrate on the neck and shoulders. Imagine you are ironing the shoulders, using the heel of your hand to roll forward over the shoulder from the back to the front. Start from the outside edge of the shoulder and move in towards the collarbone. If you are performing the massage on someone much taller than you, use your forearm to press across the shoulder and your body weight for pressure.

7 Put both hands around the head like a cap. Squeeze, lift, and let go. Do several repetitions. You can use this movement alone to combat headaches.

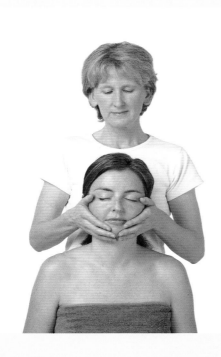

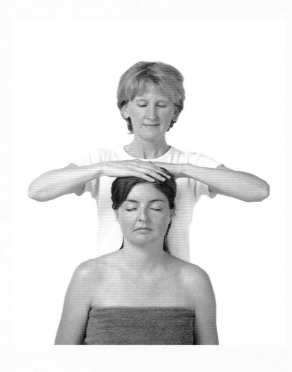

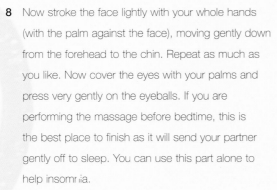

8 Now stroke the face lightly with your whole hands (with the palm against the face), moving gently down from the forehead to the chin. Repeat as much as you like. Now cover the eyes with your palms and press very gently on the eyeballs. If you are performing the massage before bedtime, this is the best place to finish as it will send your partner gently off to sleep. You can use this part alone to help insomnia.

9 If your partner wants to feel energized, finish by using a brisk rubbing motion back and forth across the scalp. Vary this with a fast scratching action, using your fingernails. Both can be quite firm and deep – gage your partner's tolerance level. Finally, press firmly but carefully on the crown, as you did at the beginning. If you can, try to leave the oil in the hair for as long as possible – an hour is good but if you can, leave it overnight (wrapped in a towel).

CHAPTER ELEVEN

marma therapy

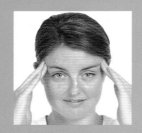

If you've never heard of your marmas, you won't be alone. Few people have any knowledge of these vital "junction boxes" of the body. In ayurveda, however, these points and areas where nerves and muscles meet are considered vitally important. If your marmas are clear and uncongested, good health follows. If, on the other hand, they are clogged (which can easily happen) you will soon start to feel under par. This chapter will turn you into a marma expert – and give some vital pointers as to how we can all help keep this hidden system in tip-top condition.

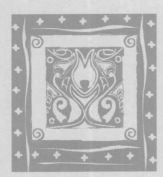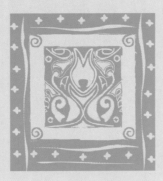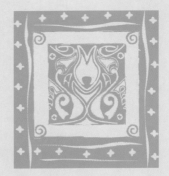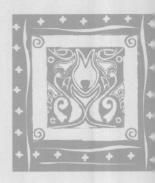

Anyone who wants to live long, appear young, and stay in perfect health should look to their marmas. Here in the West few people have even heard the word but to an ayurvedic practitioner the marmas are the key to health, emotional security, longevity, beauty – even life itself. The marmas are like the junction boxes of the body: 107 points or areas where nerves and muscles meet. While they stay clear and uncongested, you will remain healthy and happy. If they become clogged or unbalanced, you could find your confidence failing alongside your health, as both emotional and physiological functions become impaired.

The ancient ayurvedic texts describe the marmas in precise detail. Centuries of observation taught the ayurvedic surgeons that if certain marmas were cut or damaged then death, disability, loss of function, or pain would ensue. For this reason, many ayurvedic experts insist that only very skilled people should attempt to manipulate the marmas. However, there is a world of difference between attempting to manipulate the marmas of someone who has been shot by an arrow and gently pressing them in massage. Providing you don't poke and prod too hard, it's highly unlikely you will

do any damage. In the list featured at the end of this chapter I have included the effects of severe damage to the marmas (an alarming amount of premature death and disability) as a matter of interest and also a warning that, unless you are very skilled in bodywork, it is not a good idea to work too deeply!

The marmas sound, at first hearing, very similar to the Chinese acupuncture points and some people do theorize that the part of the ayurvedic texts describing the marmas was taken to China, where the theory developed into acupressure and acupuncture. However, ayurvedic physicians point out that the marmas differ in significant ways to acupuncture points. They are connected directly with the nervous system, linking the body with the brain; they lie deeper in the body than the acupuncture points; and many cover an area of the body rather than just a tiny point.

The reason why the marmas are so crucial is that they provide the link between body and mind. If the marma points are blocked, the nervous system cannot send clear messages to the brain. If there is a problem in the body, the alarm message sent from the body might simply not be able

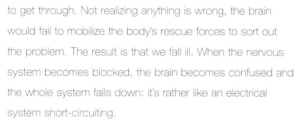

to get through. Not realizing anything is wrong, the brain would fail to mobilize the body's rescue forces to sort out the problem. The result is that we fall ill. When the nervous system becomes blocked, the brain becomes confused and the whole system falls down: it's rather like an electrical system short-circuiting.

Unfortunately, modern life is not easy on the marmas. We eat the wrong kind of diet, we don't exercise enough, we ingest and inhale vast quantities of pollutants, and expose ourselves to a bombardment of stress. The marmas valiantly try to deal with the combined debris these abuses cause but they often become overloaded and congested. When this happens we might initially suffer symptoms such as vague aches and pains; dizziness and lightheadedness; headaches; general weakness and low energy; and feelings such as anxiety, fear, and stress. If the marmas remain blocked, if the onslaught of toxicity does not ease, we are simply asking for chronic ill-health. The picture is not pretty: ayurvedic physicians warn that if your marmas are not clear you will age more quickly, your body will stop rejuvenating itself, and it will start to deteriorate.

Even more intriguing is the idea that, for some of us, our marmas are blocked at birth. Ayurveda teaches that this can happen because of something that affected us in a past life. Some people come into the world with their marmas blocked by unconscious memories from previous lives. This is the reason given for the often inexplicable illnesses which seem to be so unfair – a blameless baby or child becoming ill or suffering a chronic disease. Of course, you may feel this is complete nonsense and I'm not saying you have to believe it – but it is food for thought. Ayurvedic physicians can help to unblock the points to allow the energy to flow freely once again – providing, of course, that it is in line with that person's karma, or fate.

If you visit an ayurvedic physician, he or she will manually stimulate the marma points with either direct pressure or insistent massage. Marma therapy is certainly no feel-good massage – the pressure can be so intense you think you might bruise. When you perform your own massage and oiling techniques you will automatically be stimulating the marmas – one of the reasons why such massage is so incredibly good for you.

HOW TO KEEP YOUR MARMAS CLEAR

Fortunately there are plenty of simple DIY techniques for keeping your marmas clear. Most of the measures already discussed in this book will help them inordinately, but let's take this chance to recap a few points. In particular you should:

- **EXERCISE:** The marmas can be activated and toned through yoga. Yoga positions are designed to stimulate various points, so they automatically massage the marmas. However, any form of gentle exercise will help – swimming is particularly good.

- **HAVE A FOOT MASSAGE:** A cluster of three important points can be found on the soles of the feet. Giving your feet a gentle foot massage with sesame oil for three to five minutes a day will be beneficial. If you do this just before bedtime it will soothe the nervous system and help you get a good night's sleep.

- **EAT A CLEAN DIET:** You should already be eating a good clean diet but if not, then maybe now's the time to check back to Part Two! Acidic foods, processed, or highly refined foods can all help to clog the marmas. Remember to eat your meals slowly and calmly. It is also important to stick to regular meal times as far as possible – if you snack in between meals the food will not be properly digested and waste will be dumped at the marmas.

- **KEEP YOUR POSTURE STRAIGHT:** Good posture allows vital energy to run smoothly through our bodies. If you are slumped or slouched, your energy will become stuck and the marmas will become clogged. Yoga will help. You can also investigate the Alexander Technique, which teaches ideal relaxed posture.

- **KEEP YOUR THOUGHTS CALM AND CLEAR:** Just as bad posture can affect the marmas, so can bad thoughts and attitudes. If your mind is cramped and clogged, it will have a knock-on effect on your marmas. Practice meditation or mindfulness and try to keep stress levels down (again yoga will help).

- **FOCUS ON THE THREE MAJOR MARMA POINTS:** The three major marma points outlined below should be gently massaged every day. Use a light, circular motion, taking a few minutes at each site.

1 The major head marma, sthapani, is situated between the eyebrows, extending to the center of the forehead. Gently massaging this area with your eyes closed is good for worry, headaches, and mental strain. It will also help you sleep at night.

2 The heart marma, hridaya, is located just below the sternum, where the rib cage ends. Massaging here will help settle upset emotions.

3 Massaging vasti, the marma on the lower abdomen (about four inches below the navel), will help the intestinal tract, and ease constipation and gas.

WHERE TO FIND THE MARMA POINTS

These are the positions of the marmas as explained in the ancient ayurvedic texts. Many of these points lie within the blood vessels of the body, making it difficult for the unpracticed to locate them. They vary in size too – some are just tiny points, others spread out for several inches. It can be interesting to notice where you have pain in the body and see if it corresponds to any of the marmas. If so, you could try very gently massaging that point.

- **Talahridaya** – four points in the center of the palms and soles of the feet. This marma stimulates the lungs, and damage to it is said to cause early death.

- **Kshipra** – four points in the tendons between the thumb and index finger and the first and second toe. This marma stimulates the heart, and damage to it can cause early death.

- **Kurca** – four points in the tendons around the base of the thumb and toes. This marma stimulates vision, and damage to it can cause disability.

- **Kurcashira** – four points in the tendons below the wrist and ankle. This marma controls muscle spasm, and damage to it can cause pain.

- **Manibhanda** – two points in the center of the waist that relieve stiffness and tension. Damage to this marma can cause pain.

- **Gulpha** – two points around the ankle joints that relieve stiffness. Damage to this marma can cause pain.

- **Indravasti** – four points in the muscles around the middle of the forearm and the lower leg. This marma stimulates agni, or digestion, and the intestines, and damage to it can cause early death.

- **Kurpara** – two points in the elbow joints that stimulate the heart and spleen. Damage to this marma can cause disability.

- **Jana** – two points in the knee joints that stimulate the heart and spleen. Damage to this marma can cause disability.

- **Ani** – four points in the tendons above the elbows and knees. This marma eases muscle tension and pain, and damage to it can cause disability.

- **Urvi** – four points in the blood vessels of the middle of the upper arm and thigh. This marma stimulates the lymph channels and blood plasma, and damage to it can cause disability.

- **Lohitaksa** – four points in the blood vessels of the armpit and groin that control the blood supply to the legs. Damage to this marma can cause disability.

- **Kashadhara** – two points in the tendons above the armpit that control muscle tension. Damage to this marma can cause disability.

- **Vitapa** – two points in the blood vessels below the groin that control abdominal muscles. Damage to this marma can cause disability.

- **Guda** – one point in the muscle of the anus that stimulates the root chakra and the reproductive and urinary systems. Damage to this marma is fatal.

- **Vasti** – one point in the ligament between the pubic bone and the navel that stimulates kapha dosha. Damage to this marma is fatal.

- **Nahbi** – one point in the ligament around the navel that stimulates the small intestines and the breakdown of food. Damage to this marma is fatal.

- **Hridaya** – one point in the center of the breastbone that stimulates the nervous system, the hormones, circulation, and the transportation of nutrients, and is said to govern intelligence and a cheerful disposition. It also helps to balance movement in the body and causes perspiration. Damage to this marma is fatal.

- **Stanamula** – two points in the blood vessels below the nipples. This marma regulates blood circulation, and damage to it can cause premature death.

- **Stanarohita** – two points in the muscles above the nipples. This marma relaxes the muscles of the arms, and damage to it can cause premature death.

- **Apasthambha** – two points in the blood vessels between the nipples and the collarbone. This marma balances the sympathetic and parasympathetic nervous systems, and damage to it can cause premature death.

- **Apalapa** – two points in the blood vessels in the armpits. This marma influences the sympathetic and parasympathetic nervous systems, and damage to it can cause premature death.

- **Katikataruna** – two points in the cheeks of the buttocks that stimulate fat tissue. Damage to this marma can cause premature death.

- **Kukundara** – two points either side of the coccyx that stimulate the genital chakra. Damage to this marma can cause disability.

- **Nitamba** – two points above and out from the coccyx. This marma stimulates the production of red blood corpuscles, and damage to it can cause premature death.

- **Parswasandhi** – two points above the nitamba marmas. This marma regulates blood circulation, and damage to it can cause premature death.

- **Amsaphalaka** – two points in the shoulder blades, on the bone. This marma stimulates the solar plexus chakra, and damage to it can cause disability.

- **Brihati** – two points in the blood vessels located out from the spine, below the shoulder blades. This marma stimulates the navel chakra, and damage to it can cause premature death.

- **Amsa** – two points in the ligaments above the shoulder blades. This marma stimulates the heart chakra, and damage to it causes disability.

- **Manya** – two points in the blood vessels either side of the throat. This marma influences our sense of time, and damage to it can cause disability.

- **Nila** – one point in the blood vessel in the throat. This marma also influences our sense of time, and damage to it causes disability.

- **Sira Matruka** – eight points in the blood vessels of the neck. This marma influences blood circulation to the head and brain, and damage to it can be fatal.

- **Krakarika** – two points in the joints of the neck that release stiffness. Damage to this marma can cause disability.

- **Vidhura** – two points in the tendons below the ears that control support for the head. Damage to this marma can cause disability.

- **Phana** – two points either side of the nose that reduce stress and anxiety. Damage to this marma can cause disability.

- **Apanga** – two points in the corner of the eyes that reduce stress and anxiety. Damage to this marma can cause disability.

- **Avarta** – two points either side of the outer edge of the eyebrows that control posture and balance. Damage to this marma can cause disability.

- **Shankha** – two points on the bones between the ears and eyebrows. This marma stimulates the colon, and damage to it is fatal.

- **Utkshepa** – two points above the ears and eyebrows. This marma also stimulates the colon, and damage to it is fatal.

- **Sthapani** – one point between the eyebrows that controls the hypothalamus and body temperature. Damage to this marma is fatal.

- **Shringathaka** – four points in the palate that stimulate the nervous system. Damage to this marma is fatal.

- **Simanta** – five points in the sutures of the skull that control blood circulation to the head. Damage to this marma is said to cause premature death.

- **Adhipati** – one point on the crown of the head that controls epilepsy. Damage to this marma is fatal.

CHAPTER TWELVE

sensory therapy

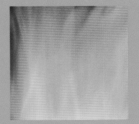

How many physicians will ask you what music you're listening to? Or suggest you drop your dreary black dress code in favor of something a little brighter? In ayurveda it's common knowledge that the colors we see, the sounds we hear and, in fact, all our senses, can have an enormous effect on our health and well-being. This chapter is an indulgent one: in it we'll look at ways to pamper each and every one of your senses (in a way that also soothes your predominant dosha). It's a whole new way of looking at (and hearing, feeling, and tasting!) the world.

Our senses are a vital part of our mind-body make-up – they are the means by which we experience the world around us. In return, the world around us affects our bodies and minds through our senses. So it makes "sense" that we should pay attention to how we stimulate or soothe our senses – a factor which is often underdeveloped here in the West.

Sometimes, if you want to tell which dosha rules a person, you only need to look at their home or workplace. I remember seeing a television "home-makeover" program featuring a bedroom painted in ethereal blues and silvers, with angels floating on clouds and a bed suspended in mid-air. It was such a vata bedroom I almost laughed out loud – particularly when its fey, airy (totally vata) owner appeared. I had an urge to phone them up and beg them to introduce a little solidity, some grounding kapha, and some warming, energizing pitta, into the room.

With that in mind, let's look at the various senses and think about how they can affect us in ayurvedic terms.

SIGHT

When you consider that everything we see will affect us, it makes sense to give particular thought to our living spaces and our immediate environment. What do you see when you look around your home and your workplace? Are they places of cool serenity or bustling energy? What colors surround you? What objects do you keep around you? Are you surrounded by clutter or clarity?

- Clutter will tend to trap stagnant prana, or energy. It will make you feel muddled and uneasy. All the doshas will benefit from a good clear-out. This will be particularly hard for kaphas who cannot bear to part with anything.

But do try to rid yourself of things you don't use – donating them to a good cause may help the process. How can you motivate yourself to clear out clutter? Vatas will usually need to see clutter-clearing as a special one-off project: just dive in and get the whole job done in one enormous burst of activity. Pittas are more organized and can cope with planning a schedule – perhaps clearing one room a week. Kaphas will probably baulk at this unless they do it slowly and carefully – just one drawer or cupboard at a time!

- Look at the objects in your home – are they solid and heavy or lightweight and floaty? If you feel a need to be more grounded, to have more balanced kapha in your life, you might want to introduce some solidity. On the other hand, if you have a kapha imbalance or an over-abundance of kapha, it might be an idea to introduce some lightness to your life – some more delicate furniture perhaps? If in doubt, aim for a balance.

- What pictures do you have in your home and office? Are they all pale soft watercolors, vibrant modern art, or heavy old masters? What kind of energy do you think you actually need around you? If you need soothing and calming, perhaps you should be looking at soft and gentle works in pastel shades. If you need "firing up" how about choosing something vibrant and energetic (children's paintings often do wonders for people who need a dose of pitta). Would you benefit from the grounding of an earthy kapha woodcut? Vatas should remember that anything too powerful will overwhelm them. The key is to put up a painting and live with it for a few days to discover how it makes you feel.

Color

What colors are there all around you? Do you always choose the same color clothes or paint every room in the same basic tone? By now, you will probably be able to work out what sort of colors you may need, based on your predominant dosha. See page 164 in the chapter on Vastu Shastra for more detail on colors.

VATA: You need to surround yourself in the main with warm colors, in soft, soothing pastels. Avoid dark colors and be careful with overly vivid shades which will upset your natural sensitivity. You will find you feel much more balanced and upbeat if you choose colors from the warm end of the spectrum – yellow, orange, and red (although in soft tones such as warm pinks rather than bright red). Gold is also a warming tone for vata.

PITTA: Ten to one you will have a wardrobe full of red (and probably also black) clothes, decorate your home in punchy colors, and drive a bright red car! If you want to cool down (in every way) plump for cool pale colors – blue, indigo, and purple tones will take off the heat. Silver, rather than gold, is good for pittas so choose silvery tones for your candlesticks and bowls, and wear silver or platinum jewelry.

KAPHA: Most colors work well for you, although you should try to steer clear of dark greens and blues which will be too watery and muddy for you. Go for bright cheering, energetic colors – and strong exciting designs and patterns. Gold is cheering and warming for kapha. You should avoid white – it will drain you – so no all-white minimalist interiors for you please!

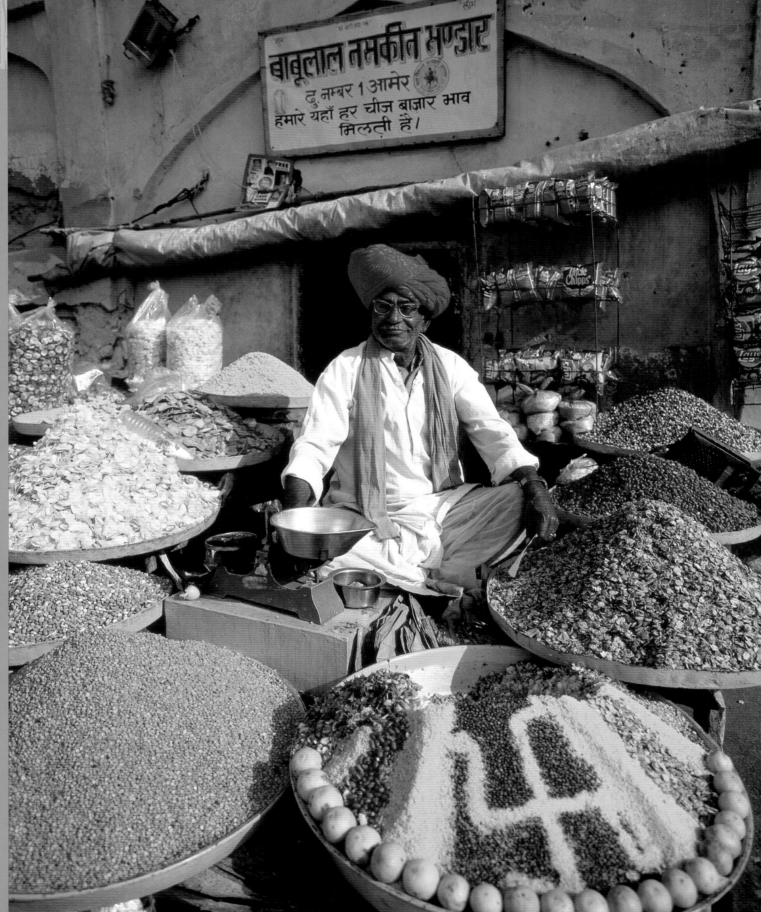

TASTE

Taste is enormously important in ayurveda. In fact the word means far more to someone versed in ayurveda than the mere sensation on the tongue. In ayurveda there are considered to be six tastes: sweet, sour, salty, pungent, bitter, and astringent. Particular tastes can balance particular doshas while unbalancing others. Let's have a look at the six tastes:

- **SWEET:** Sweet tastes give feelings of comfort and are universally liked. They help nourish the skin and strengthen bones and tissues. They soothe pitta and vata but should be kept to a minimum by kapha.

- **SOUR:** Sour tastes stimulate digestive fire and are generally good for the digestion and the heart. They soothe vata (helping vata energy move down, thus assisting with elimination) but tend to aggravate both pitta and kapha.

- **SALTY:** Salty tastes can increase the digestion and promote salivation and sweating. They are good for vata but can aggravate pitta and kapha. Too much saltiness can cause wrinkles and skin problems, and graying or balding hair.

- **PUNGENT:** Pungent tastes (eg. onions, garlic, chili, and other spices) increase appetite and promote secretions. They are helpful for kapha as they are stimulating. However, they increase vata and pitta so need to be used sparingly by these doshas.

- **BITTER:** Bitter herbs and spices such as fenugreek (coffee is also included in the bitter category) are said to have a lot of benefits, including helping skin diseases and cooling fevers. Bitter tastes increase vata so should be kept to a minimum by vatas but can be freely used by pitta and kapha.

- **ASTRINGENT:** Astringent tastes (i.e. pomegranates, garbanzos/chick peas, unripe bananas) can help cleanse the blood and soothe ulcers. Vata types should avoid if possible, but astringent tastes are very useful for out-of-balance pitta and kapha.

Start to become aware of the various tastes. Where possible make sure you have a variety of tastes in your food, boosting those which are helpful to your dosha. Notice how you feel if you do eat a food with a taste which aggravates your major dosha. Really notice the taste of the food you eat. Different tastes are detected in varying parts of the tongue – can you work out which you taste where?

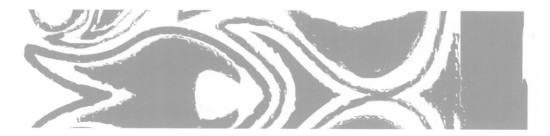
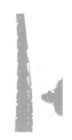

SCENT

Smell is a highly powerful sense but one we often overlook. Scents affect the limbic system of the brain and so have a direct influence on our moods. Ayurveda has recognized this for millennia and most practitioners will use scent judiciously, to influence both body and mind.

Aromatherapy is a wonderful way to help balance the doshas. You can choose an oil which has a generally good effect on your predominant dosha or pick an oil that will have a balancing effect on any dosha you may feel is out of sync at any particular moment. However, some people prefer to let their noses guide them and simply choose the oil which smells right.

- **VATA:** Soothe airy vata with cedarwood, geranium, sage, juniper, ylang-ylang, lavender, patchouli, basil, orange, and cloves.

- **PITTA:** Fiery pitta can be balanced with lavender, vetivert, jasmine, rose, mint, sandalwood, and cinnamon.

- **KAPHA:** Earthy kaphas will warm to basil, rosemary, camphor, cloves, eucalyptus, juniper and marjoram, frankincense, sage, and lemon.

You can use essential oils in myriad ways: add a couple of drops of oil to your bath water, use oil burners to scent your room, or put a few drops of an oil on a tissue and sniff through the day. In particular, vatas will benefit from having aromatherapy massage or by adding vata oils to the base oil recommended in the massage chapter on page 96. Pittas should have oils burning in a pot on their desk or in their living rooms/bedrooms. Kaphas will find it very useful to use steam inhalations: put a few drops of the chosen oil into a bowl of just boiled water, throw a towel over your head and the bowl, breathe deeply, and inhale the oil vapors.

What other ways can you introduce scent into your life? Think about the following:

- Place fresh flowers around your home and on your desk. Again, choose the kinds of scents which balance your dosha – or which you like the best!

- Keep a bottle or two of your favorite aromatherapy oils to hand alongside some tissues. If you want to shift your mood, simply put a couple of drops of the appropriate oil on the tissue and sniff.

- Scent your bedlinen with relaxing, soothing oils to help you sleep.

- Try growing flowers and herbs in window boxes outside your windows. Choose spicy, aromatic culinary herbs for your kitchen windowbox; cheering, stimulating plants (like geranium) outside your living room; and soothing, peaceful plants (lavender, chamomile, night-scented stock) outside your bedroom.

- Use plenty of herbs and spices in your cooking. Ayurveda teaches that herbs and spices have numerous healing properties, so try to incorporate the ones which help your dosha whenever you can (refer to Food Guidelines page 182).

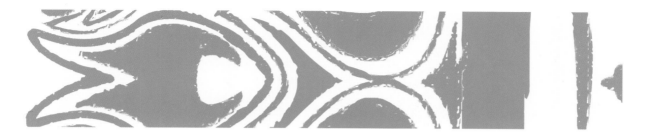

SOUND

Ayurveda puts great emphasis on the sense of hearing, and certain kinds of sacred music are played at particular times of the day to balance the constitution. You might like to find some of these and experiment with them. Equally, you might want to play with other types of music.

- Try listening to various kinds of music – soft, floaty "New Age" music is often very vata in influence but so too is some modern jazz, with its erratic, jerky energy. Music which has the punchy, dynamic energy of pitta could include rock and some classical pieces. How about kapha? Are earthy drumbeats or solid marches appropriate? How does each type of music make you feel? Try listening to different music at different times of the day and see if you have varying likes and dislikes according to the time of day.

- There are times when you don't need any sound or music at all. Sometimes silence can be very soothing, particularly for those with pitta imbalance or those constantly bombarded with noise. Make space for times in the day when you can just be quiet and still.

- The sounds of nature can be soothing, balancing, and grounding for all the doshas. Take time to sit in your garden, or go to your local park, and just listen to the birdsong or the hum of insects.

- Think about making sounds yourself. Singing (either full songs or sounds), toning, chanting, humming, groaning, or shouting might all be therapeutic at differing times – no matter what you think it might sound like to others. Do you play an instrument? Would you like to learn or start again with one you played as a child? Think about the various qualities of each instrument – which would suit or balance you best?

- If you want to go for the real thing, find a shop which specializes in "World Music" and ask for some advice on sacred Indian music.

- Some Western ayurvedic practitioners say that Gregorian chant can be a good substitute for the classical vedic music. You might like to investigate forms of overtone chanting from the Tibetan and Mongolian traditions as well. These types of music appear to be deeply healing for all types.

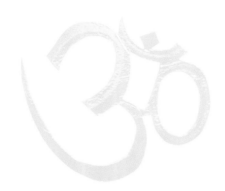

TOUCH

Touch is often the forgotten sense. This is unfortunate as our skin is incredibly sensitive and the feeling of varying textures against it can be a wonderful way of expanding our sense of body awareness.

- Become aware of various textures: take off your shoes and walk on wood, sand, grass, earth, stone. How does each feel?

- Notice how things feel when you hold them in your hands. How does a stone differ from a piece of wood? How does an egg feel or a lemon? Learn to expand your sense of touch so you pick up every nuance.

- Do certain things feel nicer than others? Why? Are there things you don't like to touch? Some people, for example, hate to put their hands in the earth. If this applies to you, you might need to introduce some grounding kapha into your life.

- Don't just feel things with your hands and feet. How does your body feel if you lie naked on different fabrics? On cotton sheets and synthetic sheets? How about silk, satin, velvet, linen, wool, fur? How does it feel when you put oils in a bath? Does the water feel different when you have a bath and when you have a shower? How do different kinds of cream and oil feel on your skin if you massage them in? How does your body feel if you brush it with a loofah or skinbrush?

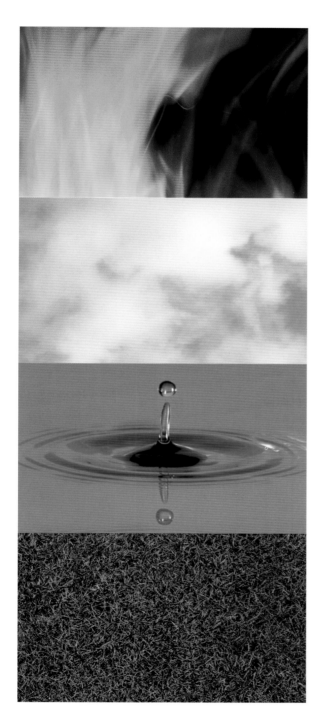

THE ELEMENTS

As you already know, the doshas are a combination of the elements. It is a good idea to try to introduce all the elements into your home – paying particular attention to those you need to increase in your life. Here are some things you might consider.

- **FIRE:** Add some pitta energy to your home with a real fire if you possibly can. If not, have plenty of candles around. Fire is energizing and stimulating. It can help you feel positive and enthusiastic.

- **AIR:** Open the windows and usher in some vata energy to stimulate lightness, airiness, and imagination. Light some incense sticks or smudge your home to purify it with the element of air.

- **WATER:** Water is calming, soothing, and gives emotional strength. Place a bowl of water (perhaps with flower petals floating in it or with beautiful pebbles in it) in your living room or bedroom.

- **EARTH:** Ground yourself with earth energy – large pebbles make good door stops; or introduce earthy ceramic bowls, stone containers, or beautiful crystals. Keep a bowl of salt on your table.

CHAPTER THIRTEEN
beauty secrets

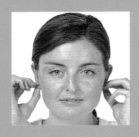

Who doesn't want to be more beautiful? In its 5,000 years of existence, ayurveda has come across some sure-fire ways to improve your looks – as well as your general health and well-being. Hoards of celebrities (who rely on their looks for their work) use ayurveda as their secret beauty weapon. It's the reason for all those perfect complexions, clear eyes, and perfect bodies (well, okay, genetics may play a part but ayurveda certainly plays a supporting role). There's no reason why you shouldn't follow where they lead and in this chapter you'll discover just how to do it.

In ayurveda, health and beauty are just two sides of the same coin. By following ayurvedic guidelines you will automatically find your skin improving and your hair becoming more lustrous. In addition, your body weight should naturally adjust itself to the optimum.

Spending time on beauty is not considered vain or time-wasting in ayurveda – it is thought to be essential time spent caring for your body and your self. Your beauty regimen should be a ritual, a small piece of "time out" for you. Look on it as a mini-meditation. Use it also as a time to appreciate your body and your face, rather than as a time to put yourself down. Look at yourself in the mirror – honestly. Yes, there will be parts of yourself that aren't perfect because absolutely nobody is perfect. It would be a boring world if we were all symmetrical and bland beauties. Just remember that even the so-called supermodels have parts of themselves they don't like, ridiculous though that may sound. Start by finding one part of your body you don't mind as much as the other bits. Gradually try to increase your "okay" quota.

If you still can't bring yourself to like your body, at least accept that it does a wonderful job for you. Your eyes give you the chance to see the world around you, your ears allow you to hear, and your nose gives you the ability to smell. Your hands are wonderful tools – without them, where

would you be? Your feet and legs carry you around, so remember, before you condemn yours out of court, that there are people confined to wheelchairs who would love the use of a pair of legs (whatever their shape or size). Yes, your bum may be big but life would be very uncomfortable without it, wouldn't it?

Do you get the picture? Your body is a wonderful creation and you should take every opportunity to appreciate it. Love it, care for it, pamper it, spend time on it.

Ayurvedic beauty is not expensive. In fact, it's totally the opposite. There's no need to spend a fortune on fancy cosmetics – you don't need fifteen different creams and ointments; in fact you don't need to buy much at all. Ayurvedic beauty simply asks that you cleanse, nourish, and moisturize your skin. There are now many companies producing ayurvedic products specifically for each dosha. Alternatively, you could make your own products quite simply at home. Ayurveda takes a practical approach to beauty by using mainly storecupboard ingredients.

Whatever you choose, one thing is vital: don't rush your beauty regimen. Use it as a time for quiet mindfulness, akin to meditation. Mindful beauty regimens help to provide small oases of calm in a hectic day – an opportunity for a few moments of peace and a tiny de-stressing treatment. In ayurveda, beauty really is far more than skin deep.

HOW TO DISCOVER YOUR AYURVEDIC SKIN TYPE

You probably already know your predominant dosha by now, and your skin probably fits into the picture well. But let's just recap, looking specifically at how the three doshas show themselves in your face and skin. Look at yourself closely in a mirror – you may find your skin is actually rather different from how you imagine it.

VATA

- your skin feels dry, rough, cold, and has a thin quality
- your skin is bluish in tone
- you have small, fine pores
- your skin easily lines and your veins may be very prominent (particularly noticeable on your neck and hands)
- your skin easily gets dry and chapped, particularly in cold weather

PITTA

- your skin feels warm or hot, soft and slightly oily
- your skin is reddish in tone
- your pores are generally small and fine but they are larger on your T-zone (forehead, nose, and possibly chin)
- you tend to have freckles or moles and sometimes broken thread veins
- your skin burns easily in the sun

KAPHA

- your skin feels cool, oily, moist, and has a thickness to it
- your skin is yellowish in tone
- your pores are generally large and open all over your face
- you tend to have problems with oiliness and blackheads

THE ROUTINE

The routine for each dosha is much the same. You should cleanse, massage, and moisturize your skin in the morning when you get up and again in the evening, before bed. Your basic beauty ritual should take roughly ten minutes.

CLEANSE AND REFRESH

If you are wearing make-up, remove it using softened ghee (see page 197 for recipe). If the ghee is solid, simply put it in a bain marie (in a bowl placed over a pan of hot water) until it melts. Use small circular movements to remove all vestiges of make-up. If you don't like the smell of ghee you can use a little oil (sesame for vata, coconut for pitta, tiny bit of sunflower for kapha).

Now splash your skin with rosewater or plain cold water to hydrate and refresh it.

MASSAGE AND MOISTURIZE

Now you can perform the most essential part of your routine – facial massage. At first this routine will seem fiddly and take quite a while but do persist – it will soon become second nature and need not take long at all. It is absolutely wonderful for your skin, nourishing and moisturizing it at the same time.

The oil you choose will depend on your skin type: sesame oil for vata skin, coconut for pitta, and sunflower for kapha. Massage the face using a very gentle stroke. Do not scrub, or rub up and down as this stretches the skin.

1 Starting at the top of the nose between the eyes, use your thumbs and index fingers (no oil) to pinch gently but firmly all along each eyebrow. Continue as far as possible along the temples, towards the tip of each ear.

2 Using the same pinching movement, start from the center of the chin and this time work slowly along the jaw-line and up to the base of the ear. Repeat steps one and two three times.

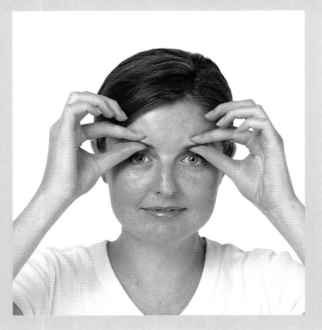

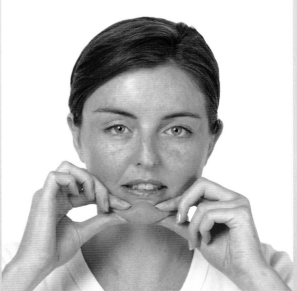

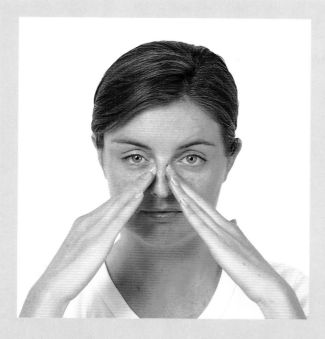

3   Dampen your skin with a wet cloth. Now dip your fingers lightly in the oil and rub your palms together to get an even spread of oil. Sweep up either side of your nose, from chin up to forehead and then down either side of your cheeks (as if your hands were tracing the lines of a fountain).

4   Place your fingers at the top of your nose and slide them up to the top of your forehead three times. Now take your fingers out from the center of your forehead to the edges of the forehead, by the hairline. Do this three times too.

5   Make small spiralling movements all over your forehead, using the pads of the first three fingers. Move horizontally to the hairline and vertically up into the hairline (avoid your hair if you aren't planning to wash it). Pay particular attention to the temples.

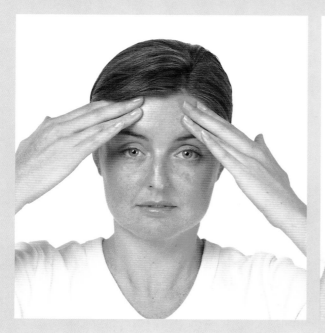

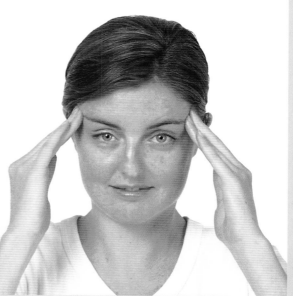

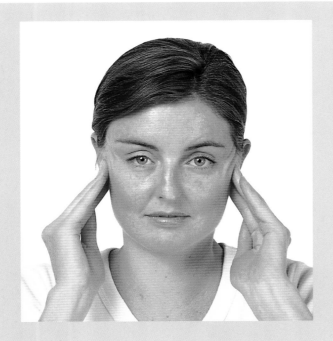

6 Now work on the sides of your face, spiralling your fingers from the end of your eyebrows out to your ears. Follow the same procedure, using smooth, sliding movements. Now take your fingers down the face to the edge of the eyes and follow the same moves out to the ear again.

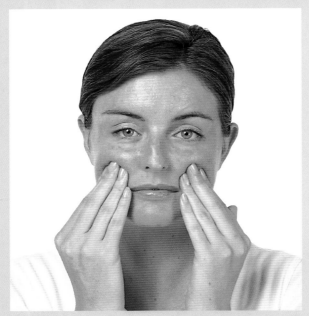

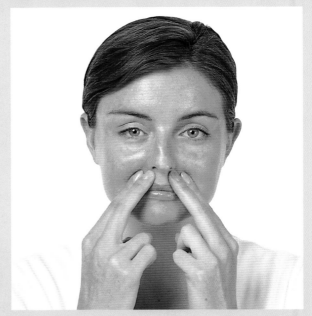

7 Now work over the middle area of your face using spiralling and sliding movements, working from below the eyes out to the sides of the face.

8 Next take your fingers from below the nostrils down to the edges of your mouth. Repeat from the nostrils to the lower part of your jaw. Once again you are first spiralling, then sliding and stroking.

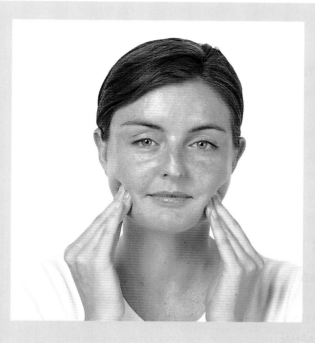

9 Work around your jawline with small circular movements
– you can press more deeply here, but still be gentle and
don't pull your skin.

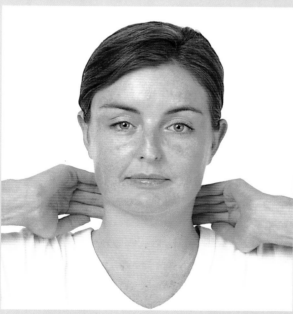

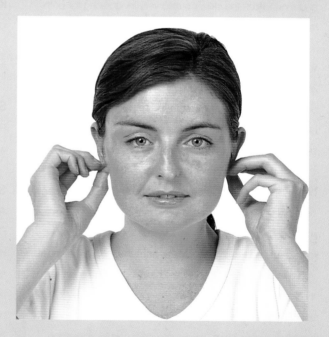

10 Massage all around your neck, using circling movements
and then long stroking movements, working from the
base of the neck up to the hairline. Spend a little time
rubbing your shoulders to release tension.

11 Pinch all around the outer edges of your ears. Give your
lobes a few swift tugs. Wiggle your finger around the
inside of your ear, but don't go too deeply.

5

soothe your soul

CHAPTER FOURTEEN
nature therapy

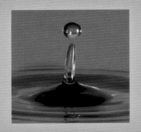

Nowadays the vast majority of us are quite divorced from nature. We can barely distinguish one tree from another and, in our centrally-heated, air-conditioned homes and offices we are hardly even aware of the passing seasons. Ayurveda can redress the balance and put us back in touch with the world around us. Our bodies and minds are still, at a deep level, attuned to the natural world and by working with the seasons and the healing power of nature we can bring ourselves back to balance.

As you will know off by heart now, ayurveda is truly holistic. Everything in life affects everything else. So it's not altogether surprising that ayurveda should teach that shifts in the weather, the ever-turning cycle of the year, should cause shifts in our own bodies and minds. The three doshas rise and fall as the year turns, each having their own periods of predominance and decline. Of course, this affects the balance of the elements within ourselves and, if we are not prepared, we can easily slip into imbalance. This means that you need to take especial care during those times of the year in which your predominant dosha is dominant.

By learning how to notice these shifts, and adapt ourselves accordingly, we can become balanced and in harmony, not just with ourselves but with nature itself. In ayurveda, this process of shifting lifestyle according to the seasons is so important, it has its own name: ritucharya. Don't panic – it doesn't mean you have to overturn your entire lifestyle every few months; rather that you need to become aware of the shifts in the seasons and move the emphasis of your diet and activities accordingly. In India it is a natural way of life: made simpler by the fact that food is eaten seasonally.

If you visit an experienced ayurvedic physician he or she will give you precise guidelines for what to do and eat at each season. Here we only have space to give you very general pointers. Because of this, some of the suggestions may seem contradictory to your individual doshic guidelines. You don't have to follow them religiously: use them as general pointers – i.e. everyone should have more warming food in winter and more cooling food in summer (whatever your predominant dosha).

If you find the food advice given here too confusing, stick to the guidelines for your predominant dosha and just follow the other hints. However, if you feel confident with your ability to detect which foods your body wants and needs you may like to fine-tune your diet with these additional pointers. Try them out and see how they affect your well-being. Where certain strategies can be particularly difficult for certain doshas, these are highlighted. Let's have a look at the kind of things we should be looking out for in each season:

SPRING

In early Spring kapha energy holds sway but soon starts to shift and liquefy as the days get warmer and life starts to burst out all around us. Spring is mainly warm, moist, and "unctuous" (oily). You need to take care at this time to avoid going down with spring colds and coughs, allergies, and hay fever.

- At the beginning of spring (while the days are still cold) you will mainly be following the guidelines for winter. As it gets warmer and drier, shift to summer guidelines. Use your intuition and common-sense to work out what you need.

- Get up early and enjoy the fresh energy of morning. Go for a walk and enjoy nature. You might like to do your Sun Salutations outside or practice your yoga under a tree.

- Your diet should become lighter as the days become lighter, turning away from heavy, oily, sweet foods (which aggravate kapha energy) and choosing lighter, fresher foods such as fresh vegetable soups (bitter tastes such as spring greens and spinach are excellent now) and

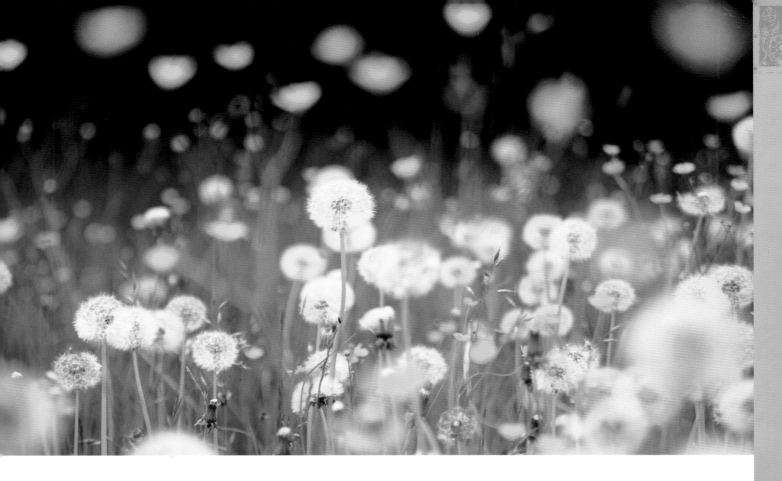

light stews with barley and rice. Even if your dosha can cope with them you should steer well clear of dairy produce, cold drinks, and ice cream. Cut down on your use of ghee. It's okay to eat meat but stick to chicken, turkey, and venison (providing your dosha allows them). Use hot spices such as ginger, cayenne, black pepper, and chili – but don't overdo them if you have a strong vata or pitta constitution.

- A cup of hot water with a teaspoon of honey can help balance kapha energy. Ginger and cinnamon tea is also great at this time of year but be wary if you have strong pitta in your constitution.

- This is an excellent time to undergo a detox – in ayurvedic terms this is known as panchakarma. Don't go for a total fast; instead consider short juice fasts (apple or pomegranate juices are ideal), or a week when your diet consists of alkaline vegetables and juices (and no coffee, tea, alcohol etc!) Alternatively, follow the guidelines for a short weekend detox given on pages 171–177.

- Start to exercise more – and more vigorously.

- Have plenty of massage using warming sesame oil (if you are a very hot pitta, stick to your usual oil).

- Don't be tempted to have a daytime nap at this time of year – it will make you feel muggy and unrested.

SUMMER

As the sun becomes hotter, pitta energy rises. This is a time when anyone with strong pitta energy should be very careful as pitta can easily become unbalanced, causing indigestion, stress etc. However, pitta energy can make anybody overheat. The key concept is to keep your cool.

- Start the morning by rubbing coconut oil into your skin before having your morning bath or shower. Coconut is cooling and soothing. If you are a very chilly vata you should skip this.

- In the main, your diet should consist of colder, sweeter, softer foods, and cool drinks (unless you are strongly vata). Cold soups, salads, ice creams are all ideal summer fare if you tend to overheat – but they do tend to dampen agni, the digestive fire, so don't eat them as part of a larger meal. Avoid very hot and pungent foods – this isn't the time for searing hot curries. If you have a balanced constitution and it is very hot follow a pitta-pacifying diet (see pages 184–185). Salads are great for lunch but lightly cooked food is best for the evening meal – try Kichadi, a light, pleasant meal (see page 198). Steamed vegetables and rice are good too. Keep your meat intake down – some chicken, turkey, or shrimp once a week (if your dosha allows). Avoid red meat (even if your dosha allows it) as it is heat-inducing.

- Keep your alcohol intake down as far as possible. If you must drink alcohol, water it down (think of white wine spritzers, clear spirits such as vodka or gin diluted with plenty of mixer, or drink low gravity beers and lagers).

Pittas should try to avoid alcohol as much as possible. Ideally, stick to water and the yogurt drink Lassi (see appendix page 197).

- Your exercise regimen needs to be relaxed now so take it easy and enjoy only light, moderate exercise. Don't overdo it. Shift to cooling activities such as swimming and surfing.

- You can, however, continue with your yoga practice. Avoid inverted postures such as headstands and shoulder stands which can aggravate pitta energy.

- Wear light, loose-fitting comfortable clothes. If the weather is very hot, avoid shorts and skimpy tops and wear long but loose clothes that will protect your skin from the sun's harmful rays. Cotton or silk fabrics are ideal. The best colors to choose are white, gray, pale blues, purplish shades, and greens – unless you are a particularly chilly vata. Avoid warm colors (red, orange, and yellow) and black, as they will retain the heat and aggravate pitta energy. Wear a wide-brimmed hat to keep the sun off your face.

- Keep your jewelry simple and wear silver rather than gold. A necklace of sandalwood beads can be cooling. So too would be a pearl or moonstone necklace or bracelet. If you're a chilly vata, stick to gold.

- Keep your home and work environments cool and airy – have your windows open wherever possible. Ayurveda teaches that moonlight is highly beneficial during the hot pitta period, so keep your windows open or sleep under the moon in the open.

- Don't sit out in the sun – it not only ages the skin but aggravates pitta energy.

- Do have a rest at some point during the day – not necessarily a nap, but it won't hurt if you do doze off.

- Have a cool bath at least once (ideally twice) a day. If you can, it's even better to cool off in a natural form of water – a lake or pond, river, or sea.

- Continue to have massages using cooling oils such as coconut (unless you are strongly vata and already cold – then use your usual oil).

- You can go to bed later in the summer as it gets dark so much later – 11pm or midnight is fine. If you find it hard to sleep at night because of the heat, give yourself a gentle head massage with coconut oil and also massage some of the oil into the soles of your feet. Put a couple of drops of sandalwood oil on a tissue and keep it next to you as you sleep. You could also try sleeping on your right side.

FALL/AUTUMN

This season is considered to be dry, light, windy, cold, and rough – all attributes which aggravate vata energy. Your aim at this time of year is, therefore, to pacify and soothe vata energy. Sometimes pitta energy can still be strong too.

- Start your day early – ideally around 5am. Spend some time in quiet thought or contemplation while the world around you is still asleep.

- Continue with your yoga, incorporating plenty of bending and twisting postures. Make sure you keep up your practice of the sun salutation. Are you building up your repetitions? Build up slowly but do keep extending yourself.

- Alternate nostril breathing (see page 62) is excellent at this time of year.

- Before you have your morning bath or shower give yourself a swift massage with warm sesame oil – it will help to pacify vata energy. You may already be doing this as part of your daily routine – great! If not, this is a good time to try to fit it in, even if it's just for the next couple of months.

- Your diet should consist mainly of foods which are sweet, astringent, and bitter. Foods should still be light so avoid excessive use of fats and oil. If you are quite balanced, all doshas can follow the vata-pacifying diet on pages 182–183: think about oatmeal or creamed rice for breakfast; and soups and stews made with ghee, vegetables, rice, and lentils for lunch and dinner. Avoid salads, which are too cooling.

- Herbal and spice teas come into their own now. In particular try to wean yourself off coffee and tea and instead try coriander, fennel, cinnamon, clove, and ginger teas (experiment with a number of these to find which you like the best). Choose ones which best suit your dosha.

- Drink lots of water, particularly fresh spring water.

- Milky drinks are soothing, particularly if prepared with honey or sugar. Almond milk is fortifying and relaxing. Give yourself the comfort of a cup of warm milk at bedtime – simply heat until it starts to boil then allow to cool slightly and add a pinch each of ginger and cardamom.

- Continue to be careful if it is hot and sunny. Equally, watch out for cold spells and windy gusts – protect your head and ears from the wind, which can aggravate vata energy. Good colors for this season are red, yellow, and orange which all pacify vata energy. White can work too but may be problematic for some people, particularly extreme vatas.

- Avoid naps during the day. A short afternoon nap is okay if you're a vata constitution.

- Loud music can upset vata energy so keep your musical choices softer and quieter. Equally, try to take life at a measured pace – don't rush around or drive too fast or vata will get jumpy.

- Try to get to bed by 10pm.

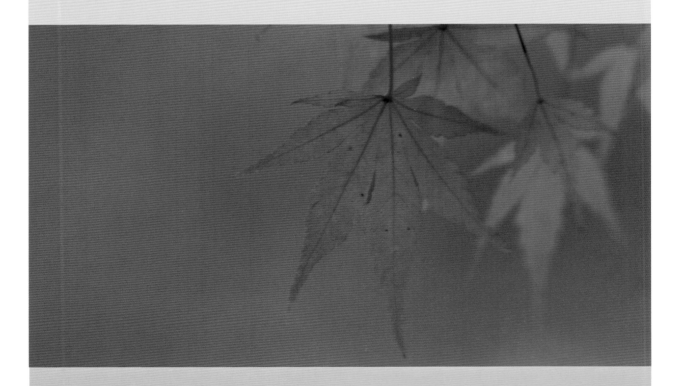

WINTER

In ayurvedic terms, the winter season is cold and dry – both qualities of vata. However, kapha qualities are here too – dampness and heaviness make life more sluggish. It's important to keep warm and well-nourished.

- The strict ayurvedic early rising is relaxed in winter so it's fine to get up around 7am. Don't race – take it easy.

- Keep up with your sun salutations in winter – it's good to remember the sun even if you can't see it! Shoulder and head stands (if you can do them) are good in winter; so too are any postures which help to open up the chest and throat (ask your yoga teacher for examples).

- Warm sesame oil will help warm your body. Give yourself a massage before bathing or showering. If you are strongly pitta and hot even in winter skip this.

- Food should be eaten warm in winter, and it's also a good idea (if you can accustom yourself to it) to drink your water warm too (it's wonderful for loosening and helping to eliminate toxins).

- You can take far heavier food at this time of year and more oil and fat, but be careful not to aggravate kapha energy. However, equally, very light foods will aggravate vata energy. Think about whole-wheat bread, hot soups made with ghee (only a little if you are strongly kapha), and stews made with vegetables and chicken or turkey. If you do like to eat meat, this is the time to do it as your agni is strong. Do observe, however, how it suits you if your doshic guidelines usually say to shun it. Even better news (for some people) is that a glass of red wine is also recommended to improve circulation and digestion. It is best to drink it before or after your dinner.

- Make sure you wear enough warm clothes – lots of light layers can be good. Don't let yourself get cold and make sure you don't sit or sleep in draughts. Always keep your head, neck, and ears covered when outdoors.

- Clothe yourself in bright, cheery, warming colors – reds and oranges are ideal. That doesn't necessarily mean head-to-toe coverage – even if you're wedded to dark gloomy colors, you can still brighten things up with a vivid scarf or sweater. Once again, if you are strongly pitta and hot you may need more cooling colors.

- Make sure you have plenty of people around you – it's a season when it's easy to become lonely or depressed. Make an effort to see people, have them round for supper, or go out to the theatre etc.

- Don't be tempted to nap during the day as this increases kapha energy.

- It's not considered a good idea to bathe in the evening although a warm shower is okay.

- You can and should undergo quite vigorous exercise at this time of year.

- Ayurvedic physicians often prescribe plenty of sex during this season!

CHAPTER FIFTEEN

spiritual therapy

Prosaic Western minds might want to overlook this chapter. After all, why bother with prayer and esoteric rituals when you can spend your time on more practical things like diet and exercise? Yet an ayurvedic physician considers your soul just as important as your body and mind. Remember too that ayurveda views everything in life as containing soul or divine intelligence, so what we tend to think of as inanimate objects (such as crystals) actually contain divine essence. There are a whole host of mystical cures which have very definite, practical effects. In this chapter we will take a look at the ones which can be adapted most easily to Western life.

CRYSTAL, METAL, AND GEM THERAPY

In the West the therapeutic use of crystals and gemstones is not generally taken seriously. It is considered just too "New Age" and flaky. Yet thousands of years of experience have persuaded ayurvedic physicians that these stones really can have noticeable effects. In the East the choice of an appropriate gemstone is treated with great gravity – a highly experienced astrologer or physician will select the correct stone, taking into account your horoscope, your psycho-physical make-up, the illness you are suffering, and your karmic history. It's not just the type of stone which is important but the actual gem. The following list offers some very general guidelines.

Note

Before you wear a stone or gem you should purify it so it shakes off the vibrations of anyone else who has held it or worn it. You can do this by placing it in salt water for 48 hours.

CHOOSING A METAL

- **GOLD:** Gold strengthens the heart, increases stamina, and is generally warming and comforting. It is therefore well suited to those of vata and kapha dosha but not so good for pitta. It is said to improve the memory and help ease stress, tension, and arthritis.

- **SILVER:** Silver is cooling, so it's ideal if you have a lot of pitta in your constitution. It can also balance vata, as it provides extra strength and stamina. Wear silver if you suffer from hot conditions such as hot flushes, heartburn, or IBS; or if you need to stem profuse bleeding (i.e. during very heavy periods). If you've had a fever or are particularly hot, silver can help cool you down.

- **COPPER:** Copper soothes excess kapha and so can be helpful if you're overweight. It is also said to be useful if you suffer from liver, spleen, or lymphatic problems. If you can find a cup made of copper, use it for your drinking water.

- **IRON:** Iron helps the bones and also strengthens the spleen and liver. It is said to be rejuvenating, and boosts muscles and nerves.

CHOOSING A STONE

- **AMETHYST:** A gem which is said to help you control your emotions. It is good for those with vata or pitta imbalance. It is also said to bring prosperity and boost clarity of thought.

- **DIAMOND:** A powerful stone, so it's not surprising that we tend to choose it as a popular engagement or anniversary ring. It is said to help rejuvenation; to be spiritually uplifting; to bring prosperity; to help foster close loving relationships; to promote romance and sensuality; and to support the heart, the brain, and the entire body. The color of the diamond is important – a reddish hue will stimulate pitta energy, a blue tone will calm pitta but increase kapha, and a clear diamond will soothe pitta.

- **EMERALD:** A stone of prosperity and communication. Emerald can help soothe nervousness and is very calming for both vata and pitta. It is also a very spiritual stone – ideal for anyone on a spiritual path.

- **JADE:** Another communicative stone, jade is supposed to boost longevity and bestow success. It is also said to strengthen eyesight.

- **LAPIS LAZULI:** This beautiful stone is soothing and strengthening. It soothes vata and pitta and can help heal feelings of fear, anxiety, and depression. It is another good stone if you are trying to become more spiritual in everyday life, as it heightens the spiritual vibrations around you.

- **ONYX:** A good stone for older people, onyx promotes memory, peace, loving relationships, and strengthens both body and mind. It should be set in silver.

- **OPAL:** The opal is a spiritual stone which can help improve intuition. It can also support your eyes, reproductive system, nerves, and head. It calms pitta and can be very useful if you are prone to migraine.

- **PEARL:** Pearls are soothing and balancing for all the doshas although, as they are linked with moon energy, they are particularly good for soothing and cooling pitta. They help to bring peace and a sense of well-being and calm tranquility.

- **RUBY:** Warm and red, the ruby is linked with the sun and so is eminently suitable for vata and kapha types. It is another stone linked with prosperity and is said to strengthen the heart, to improve concentration, and boost intelligence.

- **SAPPHIRE:** Most people think of sapphires as blue but there is also a yellow sapphire. The blue stone (curiously) is said to soothe kapha and vata while stimulating pitta. It can help ease arthritis and boost the skeletal system in general, and is strengthening for muscles. Many vedic astrologers warn that it should not be worn with diamonds, as this will create disharmony. Yellow sapphires, on the other hand, are very stabilizing and grounding – they are soothing for vata and pitta, but slightly aggravating for kapha. They are said to bring wisdom and to strengthen the heart, kidneys, and lungs.

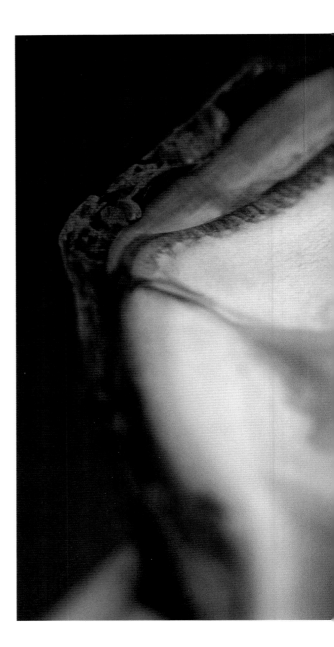

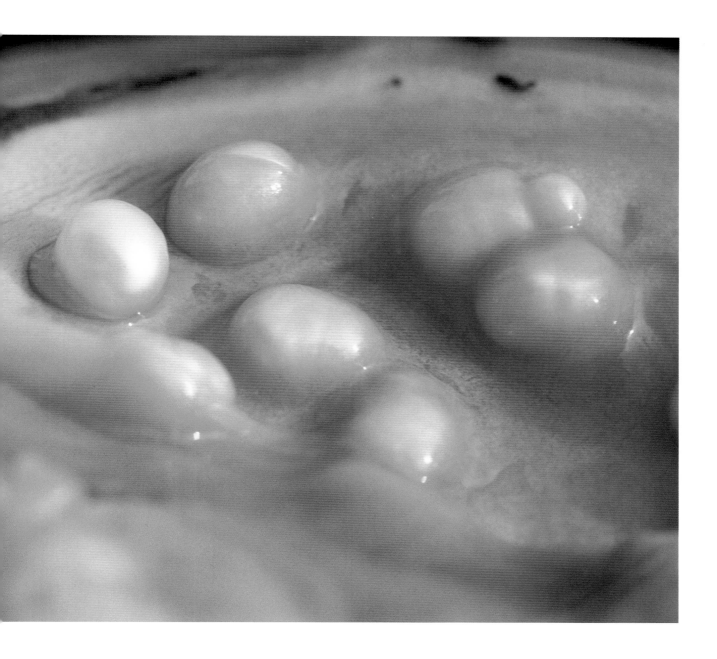

THE POWER OF PRAYER

A traditional ayurvedic physician will often suggest particular prayers and rituals to help boost healing and harmony. Here in the West, where orthodox religion is often regarded with skepticism or downright disbelief, this may seem like something to avoid. Yet there is really nothing to fear from prayer. And maybe, just maybe, by not praying we're missing out on something. Psychologists have been investigating the "science" of prayer and coming up with some remarkable findings.

Recent research has shown that prayer can significantly help AIDS patients. A study reported at the American Psychosomatic Society in Florida divided 40 equally ill patients into two groups. The group receiving prayer did not know that volunteers from ten religions and healing traditions were praying for them for an hour a day for a week. After six months, the group who were prayed for had spent an average of ten days in hospital compared to 68 days for the control group. Those receiving prayer also reported a decrease in emotional distress.

It doesn't matter how you pray, or to whom or what you pray. It seems it's the focus that is important – bringing your attention to the possibility of the divine in your life. But for many people prayer seems too much like, well, prayer – particularly if long boring periods of kneeling and hand-clasping were foisted on them as a child. If this is how you feel, try a slight twist on conventional prayer: prayer-walking. In many ancient monasteries, monks paced complicated labyrinths to focus their minds on their devotions – but you don't really need any props to prayer-walk. Simply plan a minimum of half an hour for your devotions: five minutes to focus your thoughts, at least twenty for the walk itself, and another five to sift through what you've learned. Walk at a pace that's comfortable but keep up a good rhythm. How you pray is up to you: if you have a religious faith you might want to think over scripture or recite a religious mantra; if not, you could repeat a word with significance for you, such as "hope" or "peace." You might want to use your walk to think about people who need your prayers. Or you might simply appreciate the beauty of nature around you – noticing the small things as well as the larger picture.

RITUALS FOR EVERYDAY LIFE

Another much-maligned spiritual activity is ritual. Rituals and ceremonies have become debased in our minds: festivals such as Easter and Christmas have become so commercialized and so gluttonous it's hard to uncover the original thought behind them. Children demand bigger and better toys for Christmas; they expect ever-expanding party bags for birthdays; vaster quantities of chocolate for Easter. Virtually every week there's a new card to buy or flowers to send. It all gives the notion of rituals a bad name. Yet ayurvedic physicians swear by the power of ritual and now many psychologists are beginning to agree with them.

Rituals are a lively part of everyday life in most Eastern and African countries. Here in the West, our ancestors used to follow them too. In pre-Christian times the passing of the year was marked with regular seasonal festivals in which all the community participated. By following the ups and downs of the year people got to grips with the cycles of their own lives, learning that there are times of great energy and joy alongside times of quiet introspection; times of birth and rebirth but inevitably also times of sadness, loss, and death. This knowledge was deeply healing – something we could all do with in our frenetic modern lives.

There's little use in simply giving formulaic ayurvedic rituals here. It's up to us to invent our own rituals and to make them meaningful. Start small – by sitting down as a family for Sunday lunch. Say Grace, in whatever form you fancy, to help you connect to the earth which provided your food. After you've eaten you could have a family meeting, bringing up any issues which are concerning you. If you all tend to talk at once, try using a "talking stick" so only the person holding the stick can speak. Once they finish, they lay down the stick and someone else can pick it up.

MAKING ALTARS

One small way to introduce healing, meaningful ritual into everyday life is by building an altar. An altar or shrine is a place (it might be a special table or simply a window ledge, bedside table, or even the top of the refrigerator or computer) dedicated to the sacred. It's a place you can come to meditate, pray, or simply stop and take stock every now and again. Archeologists have found evidence of altars all over the world – it seems as if building a sacred space is a very deep-seated human urge.

In India, altars are very much part of everyday life but, once again, we are not seeking to copy a Hindu altar. Our alter needs to have personal meaning for us. An altar should always reflect your own personality, your own beliefs, your own needs. If you want better health, happier relationships, greater work success, or spiritual growth, you can build an altar to that purpose. There are no hard and fast rules although, if you feel a bit unsure, you can follow these rough guidelines. Before long, I can promise, you will just "know" what needs to be on your altar.

- Candles – lighting candles and watching their flames is a way of bringing fire energy into your life. Choose a candle in a color suitable for your purpose. Green is good for healing; red for energy and passion; blue for meditation and a cooling influence; purples for spiritual awareness; yellow for friendship, communication, good luck, and wisdom; pink if you are looking for love or to conceive a child.

- A bowl of water – this represents the water element. You might like to float petals on it or put beautiful pebbles in it.

- A bowl of salt – this represents the earth element. Alternatively, you might like to use a solid stone or an earthenware pot.

- An incense holder or aromatherapy burner – this represents the air element and brings a delicious scent to your altar. Choose scents which you find attractive – many Eastern incenses are a bit too overpowering for Western noses. You could pick something that would soothe your major dosha (see page 120).

- Flowers, blossom, a potted plant or herb.

- A favorite crystal or other natural objects like stones, wood, shells.

- A statue or photo of a divinity – choose something that is meaningful for you or that appeals in some way.

- Photos, postcards, images.

RETREATS AND PILGRIMAGES

There was a time when only monks and nuns would go on retreat or pilgrimage in the West, but nowadays both activities are becoming more popular as people look for meaning and the spiritual in life. Once again – no surprise to those following the ayurvedic path – taking time out to soothe your psyche and renew your energy is seen as a very healthy and necessary practice.

How do you know if you need a retreat? Simple. Do you feel as though you just want to run away and hide? Is your whole soul, your entire being, crying out for time out? Yes?

Then you need a retreat! We all need time away from the mad, frenetic outside world. Perhaps surprisingly, there are loads of places to which you can retreat. Some are religious; many aren't. They all offer a place of peace and a time for renewal. Some are even run on ayurvedic guidelines. You might feel the need to be totally silent and mainly alone. Alternatively, you might want to just be with people you don't know – like-minded souls engaged in meditation, yoga, or giving something back to the world via community service or clearing the land. If you possibly can, it's very helpful to go on retreat once a year. A week is ideal but if this is not possible a weekend will serve.

If it's not possible to go away on retreat even for a weekend, you can always make your own retreat at home. It takes more planning and discipline but can be done. You simply have to tell everyone you are just not around, then put the ansaphone on, put a "do not disturb" notice on the door, and make sure you have everything you need before

you hide away for your retreat. Take the time to get in touch with your body – to do your yoga in an unhurried way, to eat the kind of food you know your body craves, to read spiritual material (or not read at all), to listen to uplifting music, or revel in silence. There is no prescription – just follow your heart.

Equally, you may be drawn to pilgrimage – a longer version of the prayer walk described earlier. Here you (usually) walk to a sacred place or along a sacred route. There are well-established pilgrim routes and time-honored sacred places but you don't have to follow the crowd. Remember, the whole world is interconnected so, in a way, it doesn't really matter where you go. It's your intention that counts. You can make a pilgrimage to a favorite place in nature – a hill, a forest, a spring, a mountain. You might follow the course of a river. You could equally trace steps around a city. What comes into your mind? What feels right for you? Follow your instinct.

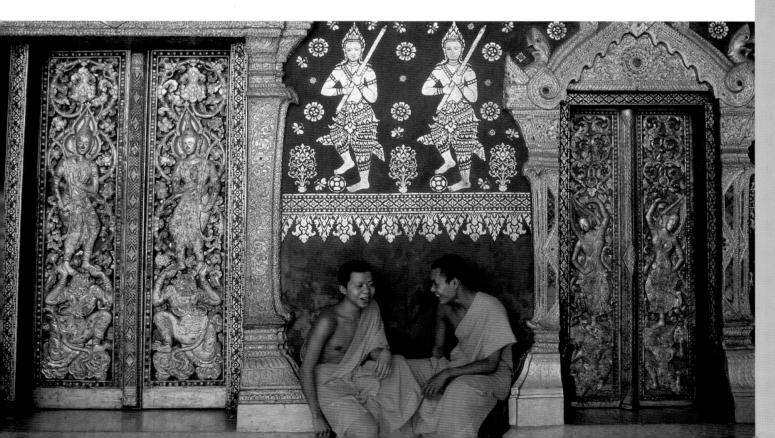

CHAPTER SIXTEEN

home harmony

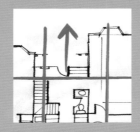

A home should be a healing space, a sanctuary to which you can retreat from the hurly burly of the outside world. Yet many of us live in homes which are far from harmonious. This can generally be easily remedied – with some clearing and space cleansing, re-arranging and decluttering. The extra-special secret ingredient you'll learn about in this chapter is the art and science of Vastu Shastra. It's the ayurvedic equivalent of feng shui and helps vital energy to flow smoothly through your living space. The result? A harmonious home with happy, healthy inhabitants.

Virtually everyone has heard of feng shui, the Chinese system of "energetic architecture" which acts as a kind of acupuncture for houses. Yet few people are aware that India has its own equivalent – Vastu Shastra.

At heart the two systems are very similar. Both argue for symmetrical buildings, for clarity and lack of clutter; and both insist that there are beneficial directions in which to site the various rooms of the house and the furniture within it. Just as feng shui has the ba-gua, a map of the various directions and the corresponding areas of life, so Vastu Shastra has a mandala or sacred diagram called the Vastu Purusha Mandala. The legend goes that a formless being threatened to cause disruption between heaven and earth. The Gods seized the being and laid it face down on the earth where it took the form of a human being (the purusha). "The mandala forms the basis for the understanding of the movement and flow of energy through space," explains Vastu Shastra practitioner Kajal Sheth, "Cosmic energy is said to enter a structure through the purusha's head in the north east, move down its arms in the south east and north west and finally gather at its feet in the south west. So to attract vital energy inside the home it is important to keep the east, north east and north clear, open and unobstructed." Once the energy has entered the house, it is important to ground it. So the ground in the south and west is traditionally kept slightly higher and has less openings, less open space, and more solid walls.

Houses that are built according to Vastu Shastra principles generally face east to maximize the amount of early sunlight entering the house. The ancient Indians observed that the rising sun with its gentle heat and light is a source of vitality, while the setting sun, in their view had far too much heat and glare. They also believed that the ultra violet rays emanating from the rising sun were very beneficial for human health.

Before building starts, an elaborate system of rituals takes place. First the land is levelled, to symbolize bringing order to a wild, unruly world. Then the land is ploughed to cleanse and purify it from its past connections. Offerings are made to appease the land, and rituals are held at precise times – during the laying of the foundations, fixing of the main door, and the owners' first entry into the house. These rituals invoke the soul of the land and convert the bare land into a living organism.

If you are planning a new home and building from scratch, it might be a nice idea to conduct your own ceremonies for appeasing the land. This might not seem as strange to your builders as you might imagine. Even in the West we still retain echoes of these ancient practices – the laying of the foundation stone, for instance, is a well-accepted tradition.

However, even if you are just moving into a (new to you) house or apartment, it can be very helpful to perform a ritual or ceremony to mark the transition. This need not be complicated. One simple ritual involves going round each room of your old home carrying a lighted candle. Pause as you go into each room and remember all the good times you had in that space; invite those memories to come with you to your new abode. Continue through the house until you have captured everything good about your life in that place. Then blow out the candle and take it with you to your new home. Light the candle in the center of the new place and invite all the good memories to come out. Then let the candle burn out. There are a few other practices you might perform.

- Introduce yourself to your new home – houses have feelings just as much as people. Tell it you will love and care for it.

- Clean it thoroughly (ideally before you move in), even if the people leaving have left it spotless. Use fresh-scented aromatherapy oils – such as grapefruit, bergamot, or lemon – in your cleaning water.

- Perform some space cleansing routines such as clapping, smudging, burning incense, or toning. The following is a very simple but effective exercise...

SPACE CLEANSING

1 Take a bath or shower. You might like to add a couple of drops of rosemary oil which is purifying. Dress in clean, comfortable clothes but keep your feet bare and remove all jewelry and your watch.

2 Go to the center of your home, close your eyes, and spend a few moments quietly breathing and centering yourself. Imagine you are breathing into and out of your solar plexus area (between the belly button and chest).

3 Light either a smudge stick or oil burner (add seven drops of lavender aromatherapy oil). If you have any spiritual or religious beliefs you can call on them to help you in your work, asking for their assistance in purifying and cleansing your home.

4 Now go around the whole space, sending smoke or the aromatherapy fumes into every room and corner.

5 Next you will need to "clap out" your home. Move slowly and steadily around your home, clapping in every corner. Clap your hands together, starting at the bottom of the wall and swiftly clapping on up towards the ceiling, as high as you can. You may need to repeat this several times in each spot – until the sound of your clapping becomes clear. As you clap, visualize your clapping dispersing all the stagnant old energy.

6 When you have finished, wash your hands.

7 Now you can go around each room in your home balancing the energy with either a bell or a rattle. Keep up a continuous ringing or rattling in each part of the room until you sense the room is clear. Imagine the sound clearing any last vestiges of old energy.

8 Return to the center of your space and once more close your eyes and breathe. How does your home feel now? Can you detect the difference?

9 Stamp your feet to ground yourself and have a good shake and stretch. It's a good idea to have something to eat and drink after this ritual.

Note

Do not perform space cleansing if you are unwell, pregnant, or menstruating, or if you feel nervous or apprehensive.

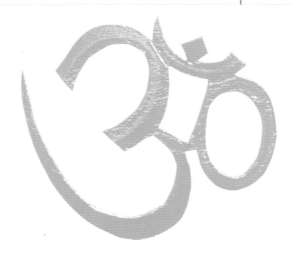

VITAL TIPS FOR VASTU SUCCESS

GENERAL

- The ideal shape for a house is square or rectangular, in a square or rectangular plot of land. Avoid triangular or irregular plots.

- The back of the house should be slightly higher than the front to contain the energy coming in from the front door.

- The front of your house should have more openings (doors and windows) than the back.

- Ideally the house should face east, to attract the energy of the sunrise. If it faces another direction, ensure that east is kept open and not blocked by trees or other buildings.

- Never have three doors in a line.

- Avoid having your toilet in the northeast.

- The central part of the house is very sensitive. Do not have a staircase or a toilet here. Traditionally it would have been an open courtyard so try to keep this area as clear, clean, and stable as possible.

FRONT ENTRANCE AND HALL

- Your front door should ideally face east and should be the biggest door in the house.

- Paint an "Ohm" symbol (see illustration above) on your front door at eye level.

- Keep the area near the front door open, clear, and unobstructed to allow the maximum amount of energy into the house.

- Place lower, lighter furniture near and around the front door. Taller, heavier furniture should be placed in the area diagonally opposite (furthest away from the door) to hold the energy down.

BEDROOMS

- The master bedroom should be in the southwest. Sleep in the southwest corner of the room with your head facing south. If south is impossible, have your head facing west. It is not recommended that you sleep with your head facing north.

- Don't let your bed touch the walls.

- Children should sleep in the west. Cots and beds should be in the southwest of the room so their heads face west. A green bulb will help enhance intelligence.

DINING ROOM

- The dining room should be a haven for relaxed eating. Paint the walls soft pink, orange, or cream.

- Install a mirror on the east and/or north wall.

- Have a rectangular dining table – avoid egg-shaped or irregular-shaped tables. Keep the dining table away from the walls.

- If possible, the dining room should be in the west of the house.

- Paintings of the rising sun and the beauty of nature (without animals in them) will create a good feeling.

KITCHEN

- If possible, place your kitchen in the southeast of the house – this is linked with the fire element in Vedic texts. Face the east when cooking. The sink should be towards the east of northeast.

- To stimulate appetite, paint the walls soft pink or orange.

- Place a mirror on the eastern wall to help strengthen finances – good food mirrors financial strength.

LIVING ROOM

- Ideally, living rooms should be in the north, east, or northeast part of the house.

- Place furniture in the south and west, allowing plenty of space in the north and east of the room.

- Put an indoor plant in a heavy pot in the south or west of the room.

- Recommended colors are white, soft blue, and soft green.

COLOR AS THERAPY

Color is considered very important in ayurveda. The colors with which we surround ourselves have a major effect on our minds, bodies, and souls. Each color produces different vibrations in the body – you can therefore balance your doshas simply with a quick coat of paint!

Colors affect people in slightly different ways. However, the following correspondences are generally held to work for most people.

RED: A very stimulating color, red is the color of blood, heat, and the heart. Red will help to stimulate the circulation and supplies energy to the nerves and bone marrow. It helps blood flow smoothly and can dilate and unblock blood vessels. It is most helpful for pacifying vata and kapha. People with a lot of pitta in their make-up should avoid red or use it with caution – maybe in small amounts such as a few red candles, a red throw, or some red cushions.

ORANGE: This warm, stimulating color promotes cheerful, sociable feelings. Orange is a great antidepressant, lifting the spirits and helping to stave off depression. It also stimulates the kidneys and can help to boost sexual energy. As with red, it's good for vata and kapha people; not so good for pittas who are usually upbeat and sexy enough!

YELLOW: A warming, nourishing, cheering color, yellow is stabilizing and makes people feel good. It has a profound effect on the glands and also activates the mucous membranes. Yellow also helps to stimulate elimination and detoxification so it's particularly useful for stomach and liver problems. As with the other warm colors, it's good for vata and kapha but should be used with caution by pittas.

GREEN: The serene, soothing, harmonizing color of nature, green calms both mind and body. It can help concentration and for that reason is useful in the office or study. However, too much green can lead to pitta disturbance.

BLUE: Cool and spacious, blue is the tranquility of a calm mind, the color of the sea and sky. It is cooling on the body and has a contracting effect. It can soothe over-heatedness and is great for pitta imbalance, particularly for sore, red, irritable skin. However, vata and kapha should use blue with caution as it is too cooling for them.

PURPLE: Another cold color, purple is considered regal and therefore somewhat remote. It has a relaxing effect on the central nervous system and can help soothe insomnia and sleep disturbances as it is slightly hypnotic. It can help to treat pitta and kapha imbalances but should be avoided by vata because of its cooling nature.

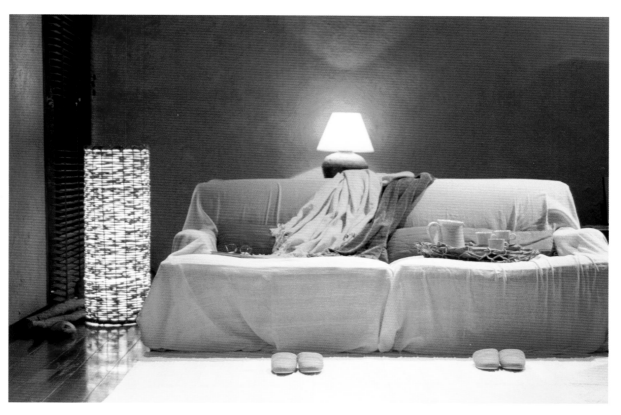

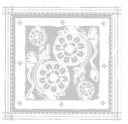   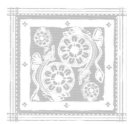

CHAPTER SEVENTEEN

ayurvedic detoxing

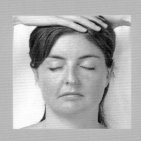

We all know when we've overdone it. We've been eating too much of the wrong kinds of food; drinking too much coffee, tea, and alcohol and generally burning the candle at both ends. It's time for a detox. Detoxing has become highly fashionable in recent years but, as you might expect, it's old hat for ayurveda. Ayurveda has been promoting periods of deep cleansing throughout its history and it has developed panchakarma (as it is known) to a fine art. In this chapter we'll look at ayurvedic detoxing and introduce a home panchakarma program which will really spring clean your system.

In ayurveda, detoxing is far more than just clearing out the body – it is considered a therapy in its own right; vital for the health of not just body and mind, but the soul too. Ayurveda's own form of intense detoxification and rejuvenation is called panchakarma. In the ancient days, panchakarma was the province of princes and kings – a potent revitalization and rejuvenation program which was taken three or four times a year. Given over a period of several weeks, its aim was (and still is) to whisk away the ill-effects of stress and pollution and restore the body (and mind) to serenity, vitality and, above all, balance. The ancient Indian physicians claimed that, with regular panchakarma, there was nothing to stop people living to 120 at least.

Modern research into panchakarma shows it really can have a good effect on both body and mind. It has found that the ghee, sesame oil, massage, and heat treatments of panchakarma loosen lipid peroxides (free radicals which cause cell damage), which are then eliminated in the weeks following panchakarma. In addition, panchakarma was found to "significantly" lower stress and anxiety, to improve cardiovascular health, and to scavenge other kinds of free radicals that cause aging and disease.

The original, traditional panchakarma is pretty severe stuff involving therapeutic vomiting, enemas, and even blood-letting – alongside more sybaritic pleasures such as oil massage and steam treatments. There are now various places in which you can undergo a modified form of the therapy – generally minus the vomiting and blood-letting – and it's a wonderful way to relax, detox, and really live the ayurvedic life.

However, if you can't afford the time or money for such a treat, you can perform your own panchakarma at home – albeit a very modified affair. It will still have a profound effect on body, mind, and soul – if you manage to follow it to the letter. The key to successful panchakarma is finding a space to have "time out" – time away from stress, strain, and the everyday mundane concerns of life. For this reason I have outlined here an "introductory" detox weekend which most people should be able to fit into a hectic schedule.

This weekend "panchakarma" is your chance to "stop the world" for a couple of days. It's simple yet still manages to be a remarkably effective way to give your body, mind, and spirit a rejuvenating break.

SIDE EFFECTS

It may seem short but even this brief cleansing break will have a deep-acting effect on your body. By allowing your body to deal only with a relatively light food intake, you give your gastro-intestinal system a rest and help to clear the body of toxic waste. For this detox you will primarily be eating kichadi (a classic ayurvedic dish which is balancing and soothing for all the doshas) and a warm fruit salad. Unlike many detox regimens, you should not feel hungry on this one as the kichadi is very sustaining. However, because you will be giving up caffeine, alcohol, and "junk food" you may find you feel a little unwell – possibly with a headache or more profuse sweating than usual. The internal oil therapy and triphala may also make your bowels a little loose. Hopefully the gentle run-up to the weekend will make these side effects negligible but I feel it's only fair to warn you that they may appear. If they are unbearable, it may be that you need to wean yourself off caffeine (in particular) in a more gentle way before undergoing this detox.

Commonly, people report they feel far more energetic after this kind of short detox. Your body will probably feel lighter and more comfortable, your mind will undoubtedly benefit too; you may also feel more mentally alert and find you sleep better or deeper.

You may notice deeper, more subtle, perhaps even spiritual, changes too. Giving yourself time like this for your body and mind signals that you are starting to care for your true self; body and soul. It can be healing on a profound spiritual level. So don't be surprised if unexpected emotions, thoughts, and feelings come up during the weekend. Pay attention to them – don't dismiss them. When we detox at the physical level, the mind and spirit inevitably follow suit.

Caution

Although this is a very safe program, there are times when it isn't a good idea to go on any detoxing program. These are:

⚜ When you're feeling ill, getting over an illness (even a cold or flu), or feel weak. You should be feeling reasonably fit and well before detoxing.

⚜ If you have any blood glucose problems or high levels of cholesterol or triglycerides; or high blood pressure. Check with your doctor or a qualified ayurvedic physician to find a way of working with this.

⚜ If you are pregnant or breastfeeding. At this time your body needs all the nourishment it can get and has other priorities.

⚜ If you are taking medication or having treatment for any condition. Talk to your doctor or ayurvedic physician before undertaking any detox or panchakarma.

⚜ When the weather is very cold or very hot – any extremes, in fact. Even a very windy or very wet period is not a good time for detoxing as the doshas will be unsettled.

⚜ If you are very young or very old. Detoxing is not suitable for children or even adolescents (unless under supervision); nor is it good for the elderly, who will not have the constitution to deal with the restrictive diet and relatively strong treatments.

⚜ Remember, if you have any doubts at all check with your physician or healthcare professional.

PREPARING FOR PANCHAKARMA

You should choose a weekend, well in advance, when you know you won't have much (if anything) to do. If you can be alone or somewhere peaceful, so much the better – if it's possible to be in the country, that's fantastic. If not, don't worry too much. Even if you can't manage to be alone, it's still possible to fit this detox around your family or friends. Explain the program to your family or friends and ask them to respect what you're doing and to allow you the time you need (and not tempt you with junk food or takeaways!) Of course, if you can persuade them to join you, it would be much easier and very beneficial for them. But don't push them – it has to be their free choice.

Try to ensure you have everything you need within your home before the weekend – you certainly won't want to go out shopping while you are detoxing. Here's the shopping list.

SHOPPING LIST

- A good stock of still mineral water
- Unwaxed organic lemons
- Ghee (you can make your own – see page 197)
- Plain cows' yogurt (if you're vata) or goats' yogurt (if you're pitta)
- Basmati rice, mung beans
- Fennel, cumin, and coriander seeds; turmeric; powdered ginger
- Apples, pears, golden raisins/sultanas, and raisins
- Fruits and vegetables that suit your dosha
- Cold pressed sesame oil
- Aromatherapy oils – juniperberry for vata, vetivert for pitta, eucalyptus for kapha. Optional others: coriander, fennel, angelica seed, rose, grapefruit, lemon
- Epsom salts
- Triphala (ayurvedic herbal preparation available from health shops)
- Optional extras: candles, flowers, soothing music, inspirational reading

appendices

food guidelines

This guide expands the brief guidelines given on pages 35-37. However, it is a guide and nothing more – as you will have by now gathered, there are many different factors which determine the ideal diet. When in doubt, ask your intuition: how do you feel after you eat that food? You might find it useful to dowse questionable foods.

DOWSING

You will need a pendulum of some kind – either a string with a weight attached or a necklace with a pendant will be fine.

1   Hold it lightly and, with your mind, direct it to move. It should start to swing backwards and forwards.

2   Ask it which way it will swing to indicate "Yes" – most seem to swing in a circular motion, usually clockwise for yes (but not always). Watch which way it swings and affirm that this will indicate "yes" from now on.

3   Now confirm which direction it will swing for "No." Usually (but not always) it will be a circular motion anti-clockwise. Affirm that this will indicate "no" from now on. Note: it doesn't matter which way your pendulum swings (it may choose to go in a straight line or do something quite different), providing it is consistent.

4   Try it out on foods you know are good or bad for you. Hold it over the food in question and ask "Is this food good for me?" When you feel confident your pendulum is giving you accurate answers hold it over foods you are unsure of.

When you become more proficient you won't even need to have the food present – but for beginners results are more accurate if you do have the food in front of you.

VATA

FRUIT
Avoid
Most dried fruits
Apples (raw)
Cranberries
Dates (dried)
Figs (dried)
Pears
Pomegranates
Prunes (dried)
Raisins and golden
  raisins/sultanas (dried)
Watermelons

Eat
Most sweet fruit
Apples (cooked)
Apricots
Avocados
Bananas
Berries
Cherries
Coconuts
Dates (fresh)
Figs (fresh)
Grapefruit
Grapes
Kiwi fruit
Lemons
Limes
Mangoes
Melons
Oranges
Papayas
Peaches
Pineapple
Plums
Prunes (soaked)
Raisins and golden
  raisins/sultanas (soaked)
Rhubarb
Strawberries

VEGETABLES
Avoid
Generally frozen, raw, and
  dried vegetables
Artichokes

Broccoli
Brussels sprouts
Burdock root
Cabbage (raw)
Cauliflower (raw)
Celery
Corn/sweetcorn
Dandelion
Eggplant/aubergine
Horseradish
Kale
Kohlrabi
Mushrooms
Olives (green)
Onions (raw)
Peas (raw)
Peppers (sweet and hot
  varieties)
Potatoes
Radishes (raw)
Tomatoes
Turnips
Wheat grass sprouts

Eat
Generally cooked
  vegetables
Asparagus
Beet/beetroot
Cabbage (cooked)
Carrots
Cauliflower (cooked)
Cucumber
Daikon radish
Fennel
Garlic
Green beans
Green chilies
Green/spring onions
Jerusalem artichokes
Leafy greens
Leeks
Mustard greens
Okra
Onions (cooked)
Parsnip
Peas (cooked)
Pumpkin
Radishes (cooked)
Spaghetti squash
Spinach (raw and cooked)

Sprouts
Squash and marrow
Swede
Sweet potato
Watercress
Zucchini/courgettes

GRAINS
Avoid
Barley
Bread (with yeast)
Buckwheat
Cereals
Corn
Couscous
Crackers
Granola
Millet
Muesli
Oat bran
Oats (uncooked)
Pasta
Polenta
Rice cakes
Rye
Sago
Spelt
Tapioca
Wheat bran

Eat
Amaranth
Durum flour
Oats (cooked)
Pancakes
Quinoa
Rice (all kinds)
Seitan
Sprouted wheat bread
Wheat

PULSES
Avoid
Aduki beans
Black beans
Black-eyed beans
Brown lentils
Garbanzos/chick peas
Kidney beans
Lima/butter beans
Miso

Peas (dried)
Pinto beans
Soya beans
Soya flour
Soya powder
Split peas
Tempeh
White beans

Eat
Red lentils
Mung beans
Mung dal
Soya cheese
Soya milk
Soya sausages
Tofu
Tur dal
Urad dal

DAIRY
Avoid
Cows' milk (powdered)
Goat's milk (powdered)
Yogurt (plain, frozen, and
  fruit varieties)

Eat
Most dairy produce
Butter
Buttermilk
Cheese (hard and soft)
Cottage cheese
Cows' milk
Ghee
Goat's milk
Goat's cheese
Ice cream
Sour cream
Yogurt (diluted and
  spiced)

ANIMAL PROTEIN
Avoid
Lamb
Pork
Rabbit
Turkey (white meat)
Venison

Eat
Beef
Chicken
Duck
Eggs
Fish
Seafood
Turkey (dark meat)

NUTS
Avoid
None

Eat
In moderation the following:
Almonds
Walnuts
Brazil nuts
Cashews
Coconuts
Filberts/hazelnuts
Macadamia nuts
Peanuts
Pecans
Pine nuts
Pistachios

SEEDS
Avoid
Popcorn
Psyllium

Eat
Flax
Halva
Pumpkin seeds
Sesame seeds
Sunflower seeds
Tahini

OILS
Avoid
Flaxseed oil

Eat
Most are suitable, especially:
Ghee
Olive oil
Sesame oil

CONDIMENTS
Avoid
Chocolate
Horseradish

Eat
Black pepper
Chili pepper
Dulse (seaweed)
Kelp
Ketchup
Lime pickle
Mango chutney
Mango pickle
Mayonnaise
Mustard
Pickles
Salt
Soya sauce
Tamari
Vinegar

BEVERAGES
Avoid
Apple juice
Black tea
Coffee and other caffeine
  drinks
Carbonated drinks
Chocolate-flavored milk
Cold dairy drinks
Cranberry juice
Cold drinks in general –
  particularly ice-cold ones
Iced tea or coffee
Pear juice
Pomegranate juice
Prune juice
Soya milk (cold)
Tomato juice
Vegetable juices (like V-8)

Barley cup
Blackberry tea
Borage tea
Burdock
Cinnamon tea
Dandelion tea
Ginseng tea
Hibiscus tea

Hop tea
Lemon balm tea
Nettle tea
Passionflower tea
Red clover tea
Red Zinger
Yarrow tea

Drink
Almond milk
Beer and wine – in
  moderation
Aloe vera juice
Apple cider
Apricot juice
Berry juice (except
  cranberry)
Carob
Carrot juice
Cherry juice
Grain "coffees"
Grapefruit juice
Grape juice
Lemonade
Mango juice
Miso
Orange juice
Papaya juice
Peach juice
Pineapple juice
Rice milk
Soya milk (if hot and spiced)
Vegetable bouillon

Chamomile herb tea
Clove tea
Comfrey tea
Elderflower tea
Eucalyptus tea
Fennel tea
Fenugreek tea
Ginger tea (if made from
  fresh ginger)
Juniper berry tea
Lavender tea
Lemongrass tea
Licorice tea
Marshmallow tea
Peppermint tea
Rosehip tea

Saffron tea
Sage tea
Sarsaparilla tea
Sassafras tea
Spearmint tea

HERBS AND SPICES
Avoid
Caraway

Eat
As many spices as possible!
Especially:
Ajwan
Allspice
Anise
Asafoetida (hing)
Basil
Bay leaves
Black pepper
Cardamom
Cilantro/coriander
Cinnamon
Cloves
Cumin
Dill
Fennel
Fenugreek – in moderation
Garlic

SWEETENERS
Avoid
White sugar
Maple syrup (okay on
  occasions)

Eat
Barley malt
Fructose
Fruit juice concentrates
Honey
Molasses
Rice syrup

PITTA

FRUIT
Avoid
Most sour fruits
Apples (sour)
Apricots (sour)
Bananas
Berries (sour)
Cherries (sour)
Cranberries
Grapefruit
Grapes (green)
Kiwi fruit
Lemons
Mangoes (green)
Oranges (sour)
Peaches
Persimmons
Pineapples (sour)
Plums (sour)
Rhubarb
Strawberries

Eat
Most sweet fruit
Apples (sweet)
Apricots (sweet)
Avocados
Berries (sweet)
Cherries (sweet)
Coconuts
Dates
Figs
Grapes (red and purple)
Lime – in moderation
Mangoes (ripe)
Melons
Oranges (sweet)
Papayas
Pears
Pineapples (sweet)
Plums (sweet)
Pomegranates
Prunes
Raisins
Watermelons

VEGETABLES
Avoid
Generally avoid pungent
  vegetables
Beet/beetroot

Burdock root
Corn/sweetcorn
Daikon radish
Eggplant/aubergine
Green chilies
Green/spring onions
Horseradish
Kohlrabi
Leeks (raw)
Mustard greens
Olives (green)
Onions (raw)
Peppers (hot)
Radishes (raw)
Spinach (cooked)
Tomatoes
Turnips

Eat
Generally sweet and bitter
  vegetables
Artichoke
Asparagus
Bean sprouts
Beet/beetroot (cooked)
Broccoli
Brussels sprouts
Cabbage
Carrots (cooked)
Cauliflower
Celery
Chicory
Cucumber
Dandelion
Fennel
Green beans
Jerusalem artichokes
Kale
Leafy greens
Leeks (cooked)
Lettuce
Mushrooms
Okra
Olives (black)
Onions (cooked)
Parsley
Parsnips
Peas
Peppers (sweet)
Potatoes
Pumpkin
Radishes (cooked)
Squash and marrow

Swede
Sweet potato
Watercress
Wheat grass
Zucchini/courgettes

GRAINS
Avoid
Bread (with yeast)
Brown rice
Buckwheat
Corn
Millet
Muesli
Oats (dry)
Polenta
Quinoa
Brown rice
Rye

Eat
Amaranth
Barley
Cereal (dry)
Couscous
Crackers
Durum flour
Granola
Oat bran
Oats (cooked)
Pancakes
Rice (white, wild, and
  basmati)
Rice cakes
Seitan
Spelt
Sprouted wheat bread
Tapioca
Wheat
Wheat bran

PULSES
Avoid
Miso
Soya sauce
Soya sausages
Tur dal
Urad dal

Eat
Aduki beans
Black beans
Black-eyed beans
Garbanzos/chick peas

Kidney beans
Lentils (brown and red)
Lima/butter beans
Mung beans
Mung dal
Peas (dried)
Pinto beans
Soya beans
Soya cheese
Soya milk
Soya powder
Split peas
Tempeh
Tofu
White beans

DAIRY
Avoid
Butter (salted)
Buttermilk
Cheese (hard)
Sour cream
Yogurt (plain, fruit, frozen)

Eat
Butter (unsalted)
Cheese (soft, unsalted, and
  not aged)
Cottage cheese
Cows' milk
Ghee
Goat's milk
Goat's cheese (soft,
  unsalted)
Ice cream
Yogurt (if diluted)

ANIMAL PROTEIN
Avoid
Beef
Chicken (dark meat)
Duck
Eggs (yolks)
Fish (from the sea)
Lamb
Pork
Seafood
Turkey (dark meat)

Eat
Chicken (white meat)
Eggs (whites only)
Fish (freshwater)
Rabbit

Shrimp – in moderation
Turkey (white meat)
Venison

NUTS
Avoid
Almonds (with skin on)
Brazil nuts
Cashews
Filberts/hazelnuts
Macadamia nuts
Peanuts
Pecans
Pine nuts
Pistachios
Walnuts

Eat
Almonds (soaked and
  peeled)
Coconuts

SEEDS
Avoid
Sesame
Tahini

Eat
Flaxseed
Halva
Popcorn (no salt, buttered)
Psyllium
Pumpkin
Sunflower

OILS
Avoid
Almond
Apricot kernel
Corn
Safflower
Sesame

Eat
Canola
Flaxseed
Ghee
Olive oil
Soya oil
Sunflower
Walnut

CONDIMENTS
Avoid
Chili pepper
Chocolate
Horseradish
Kelp
Ketchup
Lime pickle
Mango chutney (spicy or hot
  varieties)
Mango pickle
Mayonnaise
Mustard
Pickles
Salt (in excess)
Seaweed
Soya sauce
Vinegar

Eat
Dulse – in moderation
Mango chutney (sweet)
Tamari – in small amounts

BEVERAGES
Avoid
Alcohol (spirits)
Cider
Wine
Berry juice (sour)
Caffeinated
Carbonated drinks
Carrot juice
Cherry juice (sour)
Chocolate milk drinks
Cranberry juice
Grapefruit juice
Ice-cold drinks
Iced tea and coffee
Lemonade
Papaya juice
Pineapple juice
Sour juices
Tomato juice

Clove tea
Fenugreek tea
Ginger (dried) tea
Ginseng tea
Juniper berry tea
Red Zinger
Rosehip tea
Sage tea
Sassafras tea

Drink
Beer – in moderation
Almond milk
Aloe vera juice
Apple juice
Apricot juice
Berry juice (if sweet)
Carob
Cherry juice (sweet)
Cool dairy drinks
Grain "coffee" substitutes
Grape juice
Mango juice
Miso broth
Mixed vegetable juice
Peach juice
Orange juice – in small
  amounts
Pear juice
Pomegranate juice
Prune juice
Rice milk
Soya milk
Vegetable bouillon

Blackberry tea
Borage tea
Burdock
Chamomile tea
Chicory tea
Dandelion tea
Fennel tea
Fresh ginger tea
Hibiscus tea
Hop tea
Jasmine tea
Lavender tea
Lemon balm tea
Lemongrass tea
Licorice tea
Marshmallow tea
Nettle tea
Passionflower tea
Peppermint tea
Raspberry tea
Red clover tea
Sarsaparilla tea
Spearmint tea
Strawberry tea

HERBS AND SPICES
Avoid
Ajwan
Allspice

Almond extract
Anise
Asafoetida (hing)
Basil (dried)
Bay leaves
Cayenne pepper
Cloves
Fenugreek
Ginger (dried)
Mace
Marjoram
Mustard seeds
Nutmeg
Oregano
Paprika
Poppy seeds
Rosemary

Eat
Basil (fresh)
Black pepper – in small
  amounts
Caraway – in small amounts
Cardamom – in small
  amounts
Cinnamon
Cilantro/coriander
Cumin
Dill
Fennel
Ginger (fresh)
Mint
Parsley – in moderation
Peppermint
Saffron
Spearmint
Tarragon – in small amounts
Turmeric
Vanilla – in small amounts

SWEETENERS
Avoid
White sugar – except very
  occasionally
Honey – except very
  occasionally
Molasses

Eat
Barley malt
Fructose
Fruit juice concentrates
Maple syrup
Rice syrup

APPENDICES

herbs and spices for healing

Ayurveda uses a host of healing herbs and spices to soothe aggravated doshas and restore health. Many are highly specialized and can only be obtained from ayurvedic physicians or pharmacies. All herbs and spices should be treated with great respect – ideally you should always visit a well-qualified ayurvedic herbalist or Western medical herbalist if using herbs in a therapeutic manner or in large or continued doses. However, there are many safe ways of using these potent healers – in cooking and herbal infusions and teas. This is a rough guide to the properties of the various herbs and spices. You may even discover that the spice you adore and use liberally could be contributing to your problem!

ANISE SEEDS: Anise promotes digestion, so it can be helpful to eat the seeds after mealtimes. They calm vata and pitta.

BLACK PEPPER: Many ayurvedic physicians consider black pepper one of the most important spices you can take, as it is said to contain all the five elements in equal measure. Take it as a tonic in the morning after your usual morning routine. Grind seven whole peppercorns to a fine powder and mix with a teaspoon of honey. Mix clockwise, using the ring finger of your right hand. Take the mixture and slowly allow it to dissolve in your mouth. Take this tonic at the first sign of any cold or flu – or just as a daily tonic. If you want to increase your sexual energy, add about a third of a teaspoon of ghee.

CARDAMOM: This popular culinary spice promotes digestion and can be eaten after meals. It can help indigestion and travel sickness, and strengthens the teeth and heart. Peel the pods just before you need to use them, and crush the contents if necessary. Cardamom soothes all three doshas.

CILANTRO/CORIANDER: Considered to be sweet, bitter, astringent, and pungent, this herb can bring all three doshas into balance. It is very useful for cooling fevers. It also strengthens the nerves and the brain. You can use both the leaves and the seeds.

CINNAMON: A hot spice which can aggravate pitta but soothe kapha and vata. Cinnamon helps to purify the blood and can ease headaches caused by cold weather. It has anti-viral, anti-fungal, and antibiotic qualities. Taken in the form of tea, it can help to restore energy, and reduce fever and pain.

CLOVES: The pungent and bitter nature of cloves soothes aggravated kapha and pitta. They are antibiotic, anti-viral, and anti-fungal so are often used to take care of the teeth and gums.

CUMIN: Cumin is pungent and soothes vata and kapha but can increase pitta. The seeds aid digestion and purify the blood.

DILL: Pungent and bitter, dill soothes aggravated kapha and vata. It promotes digestion and can soothe sickness and stomach-ache (it used to be an ingredient in gripe water for that reason). It can help ease painful periods and soothe slight fevers.

FENUGREEK: This pungent spice is very good if you have too much vata in your system. It's used in ayurvedic medicine as a general tonic when you're feeling weak and under par. It's used particularly after childbirth when it will increase milk production. It's also worth stocking up on fenugreek if you like vata-aggravating foods and just can't give them all up at once. A little fenugreek added to your cooking will reduce the vata-aggravating effect.

GARLIC: Garlic is a wonderful cure-all, especially for out of balance kapha and vata. It is considered to be sweet, salty, bitter, astringent, and pungent – in other words it has all qualities except sour. It can be mashed up and used directly on the skin for wounds; it is also good for insect bites and stings. Garlic strengthens the blood vessels and the heart, it promotes good eyesight, and boosts the brain and nerves. It is often taken to help prevent arthritis and can also support the liver and the digestion. Try to have some garlic every day: with ghee if you are a vata, with sugar if you're a pitta, and with honey if you're kapha. If you're a pitta person, it's worth chewing some cardamom to offset the slightly pitta-aggravating quality of garlic.

GINGER: This pungent spice is very warming for unbalanced vata and kapha. Always try to buy the fresh root, rather than the powder, as it is far more effective and is now readily available. Ginger improves appetite and digestion, so encourage children who are picky or poor eaters to eat it (try juicing the root along with some orange or other favorite taste). It's also ideal for sore throats and travel sickness.

LEMON: Not exactly a herb or spice, but lemon is considered so important in ayurvedic healing it's worth mentioning here. Squeeze the juice of one lemon into a glass of lukewarm water and drink after your morning routine to soothe an acid stomach. Add a pinch of black pepper to the mixture for diarrhea, indigestion, or stomach upsets.

Lemon pickle is a cure-all for most stomach ailments. To make it you'll need 25 lemons (choose organic, unwaxed fruit) – washed, dried, and cut in half. Juice half the fruit and set the juice aside. Cut the fruit into slices (four for each half). Place all the lemon slices (both the juiced and the unjuiced) in a large glass jar, add 1oz (30g) each of ground cumin and ground coriander, and ½ oz (15g) of ground cardamom. Add a pinch of nutmeg, two pinches of freshly ground black pepper, two tablespoons of ground sea salt, and four tablespoons of sugar. Stir together well and then add the juice. Stir once more, cover, and keep in the sun (if possible, on a window ledge) for 40 days before using. This mixture will improve with age, providing you don't allow any

water (or wet spoons etc.) to touch the pickle. Take a teaspoon of pickle every day with food.

LICORICE: This sweet spice soothes vata and pitta. You can chew the root or take it infused in water as a tea. It can help soothe sore throats and ease colds. It also strengthens the eyes and nerves and can help promote good memory.

NUTMEG: This bitter, pungent spice helps to balance an excess of vata or kapha. Be very cautious with your use of nutmeg – it is toxic in large doses. However, a small pinch here and there is very useful for over-anxiety, insomnia, diarrhea, vomiting, and painful periods. It is also said to strengthen the heart. Nutmeg paste is applied externally to soothe pain and, if made with mustard oil, can cure boils.

TURMERIC: Turmeric is a pungent, astringent spice that is useful because it can soothe and balance all three doshas. Ideally, you should always buy your turmeric fresh – it is a root which looks similar in shape to ginger. It's a potent blood purifier and is soothing for a host of skin problems. It's antibiotic and anti-inflammatory in effect and so is useful for wounds. It also has a particular affinity with the breasts, so it's good for painful breasts. Turmeric is strengthening and energizing and is therefore very useful during the winter. Add it to your cooking and also take it in teas.

APPENDICES

home remedies

Ayurveda has a host of home remedies and folk cures that can be very effective. The following gives only a sample. By all means try them but do be aware that if you have a severe or persistent problem you should consult a fully-qualified medical physician.

ACNE: This is a pitta imbalance so follow a pitta-pacifying diet. Take a pitta-soothing tea three times a day, after meals: infuse half a teaspoon each of lightly crushed cumin, fennel, and coriander seeds in hot water for 10–15 minutes, strain, and drink. Try scrubbing the skin gently with a slice of fresh lime then wash off with warm water.

ASTHMA: This is generally a kapha imbalance. Try drinking licorice tea: boil a teaspoon of licorice root in a cup of water for five minutes, strain, and take a sip of the infusion every 5–10 minutes. Keep the infusion on stand-by (it can help relieve an attack – take it the moment you feel one coming on). You can also take it as a preventative measure. CAUTION – if you suffer from hypertension, only take licorice tea for emergencies as it makes the body retain sodium.

ATHLETE'S FOOT: Mix one teaspoon of aloe vera gel with half a teaspoon of turmeric, apply between the affected toes, and cover with an old sock (turmeric will stain). Re-apply at least twice a day and continue for 2–3 weeks.

BAD BREATH: This is usually a sign of toxicity in the body, generally caused by sluggish digestion. Try chewing a mix of fennel and cumin seeds (roasted together in equal quantities) after meals. Chewing a few cardamom seeds will also help.

BALDING: Pittas are the most likely to lose their hair early. To help reduce the risk, massage the scalp gently with coconut oil. Ensure you have enough calcium, magnesium, and zinc in your diet.

BITES AND STINGS: If possible, remove the sting with sterilized tweezers (run them under boiling water to sterilize), then make a paste of equal quantities of turmeric and sandalwood powders, together with enough water to make a firm paste. Apply to the affected area.

BURNS: Immediately put the burned part under cold water. If you can't get the burned part under a cold tap, then apply a cold-pack (even a pack of frozen peas will be fine). Follow this by applying the same cooling paste as for bites and stings. Anything other than a minor burn should receive expert medical attention.

CELLULITE: This is usually a kapha problem so watch your diet and avoid dairy products, candy, chocolates, fatty fried foods, and cold food and drink. Perform garshan massage (page 100). Also use a massage mix of sesame oil and mustard oil (equal parts of each) and rub firmly into the affected areas. Make sure you have plenty of exercise – walking is ideal.

COLDS AND FLU: Chills and congestion are a kapha-vata problem. Ginger is a wonderful help if you're feeling lousy. Put a few drops of ginger essential oil in a bowl of just-boiled water, put a towel over your head, and inhale the steam – this will relieve congestion. Also take ginger internally as a tea. Intersperse ginger tea with plain warm water, which will remove toxins.

CONSTIPATION: Try to keep this vata condition at bay by always pacifying vata. Fruit is a mild laxative – try eating a peach an hour after meals; pineapples and prunes are good too. As long as you're not a kapha and don't have kapha imbalance, you could try taking a teaspoon of dissolved ghee in a mug of warm milk at bedtime. If the constipation is severe, flaxseed can be helpful – boil a tablespoon of flaxseed for a few minutes in a mugful of water, allow to cool, and then drink (the seeds as well as the infusion).

COUGHS: Dry coughs are vata induced and can be relieved by eating a ripe banana with a teaspoon of honey and a good-sized pinch of freshly-ground black pepper. Repeat up to three times a day. Productive coughs come from disturbed kapha – mix together half a teaspoon each of ground mustard and ground ginger with a teaspoon of honey. Again, repeat up to three times a day.

DIARRHEA: Stew two apples until soft, add a teaspoon of runny ghee, and a pinch each of nutmeg and cardamom. Mix well and eat slowly.

FLATULENCE: This vata problem is caused by problematic digestion. Grate about an inch of fresh ginger root and add a teaspoon of lime juice. Take a good sized teaspoonful

immediately after meals. The ayurvedic herbal remedy Triphala can also be very useful.

GUM PROBLEMS: Try to find a toothpaste which contains neem oil (from natural health shops or ayurvedic suppliers). Gargling with Triphala tea can help too. Dip dental floss in pure tea tree oil and floss thoroughly.

HANGOVER: Add a teaspoon of lime juice, half a teaspoon of sugar, and a pinch of salt to a glass of water, then stir in half a teaspoon of baking soda and drink immediately. Alternatively, try taking a glass of freshly-squeezed orange juice to which you (or some other kind soul) have added a teaspoon of lime juice and a pinch of cumin powder.

HEADACHES: There are several kinds of headaches, each caused by disturbances to the various doshas. Vata headaches are usually confined to the back of the head or may start at the back and spread forwards to the front, accompanied by throbbing, pulsating pain. Massage the shoulders with sesame oil and try taking a hot shower. Ensure you've drunk enough liquid – vata headaches are often caused by dehydration. Try making a paste of a pinch of nutmeg and water – apply to your forehead and leave on for about half an hour.

Pitta headaches tend to be in the central part of the head and around the temples. They are often caused by hot sun or eating food which is too spicy. Cool yourself with a sandalwood paste: mix one teaspoon of sandalwood powder with water, apply to the forehead and temples, and leave for about half an hour. Make a tea from half a teaspoon each of lightly crushed cumin and coriander seeds, leave it to cool, and then drink.

Kapha headaches are usually associated with congestion and colds, or hay fever and allergies. Have a steam bath with a few drops of eucalyptus or ginger essential oil in a bowl of just boiled water – put a towel over your head and inhale.

HEARTBURN: This is generally a pitta aggravation. Try eating a pitta-pacifying diet and avoid all spicy, hot foods such as curries and Mexican scorchers! Cut out citrus fruit and fermented foods like pickles and vinegars. Papaya juice can be very soothing – add cardamom for extra soothing power. NOTE: ayurvedic physicians advise pregnant women to avoid papaya.

INSOMNIA: This is usually a vata imbalance. Warm a little sesame oil and rub it gently into your scalp and the soles of your feet for a few minutes. Warm, not hot, baths can help to soothe vata, as will practicing the pranayama exercises on pages 61–65. Try a warm milk drink before bedtime, with added crushed almond (some health stores sell a ready mix of almond milk).

JET LAG: Drink ginger tea an hour before flying. Jet lag is an accumulation of vata so drink lots of water while in the air and avoid tea and coffee, which will dehydrate you. When you come to the end of your flight rub a little sesame oil on the soles of your feet and on the top of your scalp to soothe vata. Drink a mug of hot milk to which you have added a pinch each of nutmeg and ginger.

NAUSEA: This is usually a pitta-related problem so avoid foods which aggravate pitta. Chew cardamom seeds, which are soothing to the stomach. Mix a cup of plain yogurt, a teaspoon of honey, and a pinch of cardamom seeds and eat slowly. If the nausea is due to morning sickness in pregnancy, try blending a teaspoon of lemon juice and a cup of coconut juice and sip every fifteen minutes.

RASHES: Another problem that is usually caused by too much pitta in the body. Melon juice can be soothing for rashes; so too can the juice from the innards of a coconut.

SORE THROAT: Gargle with a mixture of the following: a cup of warm water, half a teaspoon of salt, and half a teaspoon of turmeric. Gargle both morning and evening. You can also make a soothing tea from half a teaspoon each of fresh grated ginger, cinnamon stick, and licorice stick (crush the sticks lightly and infuse). Drink up to three times a day.

SPRAINS AND STRAINS: For sprains, make a mustard seed bag – put two teaspoons of mustard seeds in a muslin cloth – and place in a footbath of hot water. Soak the sprained joint in the water for at least fifteen minutes. You can also make a paste out of half a teaspoon of turmeric and half a teaspoon of salt (with water added). Apply to the injured joint. Support the limb with a firm bandage.

SUNBURN: Obviously it's best to avoid sunburn in the first place by keeping covered in the harsh sun. However, if you do get burned, mash up some lettuce and apply to the skin – it's very soothing. So too is coconut oil; let it liquefy over a bowl of warm water and gently smooth onto the skin. A paste of sandalwood and turmeric is also cooling but will stain the skin yellow!

APPENDICES

recipes

If you are keen to investigate ayurvedic cookery in depth I would heartily recommend The Ayurvedic Cookbook (see page 202), which is packed with information and recipes. Here are the basic recipes which are mentioned in this book, plus a few extra ideas.

GHEE

Ghee is used a lot in ayurvedic cooking, as well as in ayurvedic beauty and home remedies. It is very nourishing to the body. Ghee increases agni, the digestive fire, and strengthens every part of the body, lubricating the connective tissue and making everything more flexible. It is very simple to make as it is basically just clarified butter. You will need unsalted, fresh (preferably organic) butter.

1   Put the butter in a small pan and melt it over a gentle heat.

2   Let it reach boiling point, when it will become transparent and a white foam will appear on top.

3   Allow to bubble gently for about 15 minutes – you will know when it's ready because it will turn a lovely soft golden color and white curds will separate out from the clear oil. When the bubbling settles down and the liquid becomes almost still it's ready. Be careful not to let it burn or turn brown.

4   Filter the liquid through muslin (drug stores or chemists usually sell it in the baby department) or let it cool until the solid curds settle at the bottom.

5   Pour the clear ghee (discard the curds) into a clean glass jar (boil it first) which can be closed firmly. It will now keep pretty much indefinitely – in or out of the refrigerator. It may melt but that won't affect it in any way.

LASSI

Refreshing and cooling, lassi makes a lovely drink, especially during the summer. It is also very easy to make. Simply blend two parts of plain, live yogurt with four parts of water until creamy. You can add a few drops of rose-water if you like or some cardamom seeds.

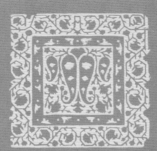
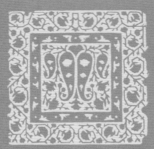

KICHADI
Serves 4

In ayurvedic cooking there is one dish which reigns supreme: kichadi. Kichadi (also known as kitcheri and a host of other spellings) is a simple rice and mung bean stew, with spices and vegetables added according to which dosha you wish to soothe. It is used extensively in ayurvedic cooking and is very simple to make. It's a soothing, nourishing dish which is balancing and stabilizing. Here's the basic recipe for a kichadi to balance all doshas.

1   Mix 1 cup/200g basmati rice and ½ cup/100g split mung beans together and wash in cold water.

2   Melt a tablespoon of ghee in a pan and add 2 teaspoons each of fennel, cumin, and coriander seeds. Cook for a minute or two.

3   Add 2 teaspoons of ground ginger (or ½ inch/1cm of fresh ginger, grated) and 2 teaspoons of turmeric, plus the drained beans and rice. Allow the rice and beans to become well coated with the ghee and then add a teaspoon of sea salt and enough water to cover the ingredients with a few inches to spare.

4   Bring to the boil then cover and simmer gently, stirring occasionally to make sure the mixture does not dry out or stick. It should take about an hour to cook.

5   If you wish, you can add vegetables according to your dosha or the season. Root vegetables will need cooking from the beginning (add at stage 3), while leafy vegetables can be added towards the end of cooking time.

The following additions to the basic recipe will help particular conditions:

- To tone the reproductive organs and promote fertility add a quarter of a teaspoon of fenugreek seeds, four neem leaves (fresh if possible), a pinch of asafoetida (hing), one onion, and a bunch of fresh asparagus.

- To strengthen the lungs add two medium sweet potatoes, one onion, four cloves of garlic, plus small amounts of asafoetida (hing), cardamom, peppercorns, and ground ginger.

- To strengthen digestion add half a teaspoon of turmeric, one teaspoon of oregano, one teaspoon of grated fresh ginger, and three good handfuls of fresh vegetables such as carrots, squash, and zucchini/courgettes.

VEGETABLE CURRY
Serves 4-6

This dish is suitable for all the doshas and makes a simple, nutritious meal. Serve with basmati rice or other grains according to your dosha.

1   Heat two tablespoons of ghee in a large pan. Add two teaspoons each of black mustard and cumin seeds, and cook until they start to pop. Now add two teaspoons of ground turmeric and one teaspoon of ground coriander, and stir in.

2   Add about 1 cup/140g each of fresh or frozen peas, chopped carrots, cubed potatoes, and either green beans or asparagus (roughly chopped), plus 2 cups/480ml of water.

3   Cover and cook until the vegetables are tender but not squashy – about 15–20 minutes.

4   Now add ½ cup/115g of plain (preferably organic) yogurt and a sprinkle of sea salt. Stir well and simmer, uncovered, for another 15 minutes.

PILLAU
Serves 4-6

This is a good standby which works fine for all the doshas, although it will particularly suit vata.

1   Heat a small amount of ghee in a pan and add 1 cup/200g of basmati rice. Stir over a low heat for a few minutes until it is well coated and glistening (but not burning).

2   Add 3 cups/750ml of water and cook until soft and tender – about 20 minutes (but check it's to your taste).

3   Meanwhile, pour a tablespoon of sunflower oil into a skillet or frying pan and heat. When it's heated, add half a teaspoon of brown mustard seeds and cook until they start to pop.

4   Add a teaspoon of turmeric, followed by 1 cup/115g of peas and ½ cup/55g of chopped green pepper. Cook for about 5 minutes.

5   Add a tablespoon of either chopped cashew nuts or pumpkin seeds (or half and half) plus a tablespoon of raisins. Now add the rice and mix well with a fork so the rice stays fluffy.

6   Add a teaspoon of curry powder if desired and salt to taste (no more than half a teaspoon of sea salt).

CUCUMBER RAITA
Serves 4

You'll find raita used a lot in Indian cookery and particularly in ayurvedic cooking. It is a great diuretic and is very helpful for high blood pressure.

1　Remove the skins from two cucumbers (preferably organic) and grate the flesh. Drain off any excess juice, place the cucumber flesh in a bowl, and set aside.

2　Heat three tablespoons of ghee in a pan and add half a teaspoon each of black mustard and cumin seeds, a pinch of asafoetida (hing), and four curry leaves.

3　Cook gently until the seeds start to pop, then add a pinch of cayenne pepper and a handful of chopped cilantro/coriander. Shake well and remove from the heat. Allow to cool completely.

4　Stir ½ cup/115g of fresh, plain yogurt into the grated cucumber. Add the cooled spices and mix well.

FRESH FRUIT SALAD

Finding a dessert or breakfast that suits all types can be tricky but this combination will work well for all doshas. However, the fruits must be as described (ripe, sweet etc.) or it won't work. Add together the following: ripe mangoes, sweet cherries, sweet apricots, sweet red or purple grapes, sweet pineapple, and fresh sweet berries.

For a warm fruit salad, stew or bake apples and pears with raisins or golden raisins/sultanas – this will work well for all the doshas and is a great breakfast for winter. You can add spices such as ginger, cardamom, coriander, cloves, and cinnamon according to your dosha.

SOLID SOUP
Serves 4-6

This soup is nourishing and filling. Soak ½ cup/115g of barley in warm water for at least two hours; strain and mix with half a teaspoon of sea salt and a teaspoon of fresh grated ginger. Put in a pan with 3 cups/750ml of organic vegetable stock and bring to a gentle boil. Simmer for an hour on a low heat, adding more water if necessary.

Chop up the following vegetables and fruits and place in a bowl: a handful of green beans, two carrots, a sweet apple, half a fennel bulb, and eight baby sweetcorn. Add a dessertspoon of raisins, a teaspoon of sea salt, a handful of chopped parsley, a tablespoon of chopped oregano, and half a teaspoon of ground cumin. Mix well and set aside until the barley has cooked (it should be fluffy and tender.) Now add the vegetable mixture to the barley along with 2 cups/480ml of stock or water. Cook for half an hour on a gentle heat.

You can either eat it like this or, if you prefer a more solid soup, liquidize some or all of it. I personally like to liquidize about half, leaving some chunky bits.

further reading and useful addresses

GENERAL AYURVEDA

Principles of Ayurveda by Anne Green (Thorsons)

Ayurveda – The Ancient Indian Healing Art by Scott Gerson (Element)

Healing with Ayurveda by Angela Hope-Murray and Tony Pickup (Gill & MacMillan)

Ayurveda – The Secret of Lifelong Youth by Karin Schutt (Time Life)

The Handbook of Ayurveda by Dr Shantha Godagama (Kyle Cathie)

The Book of Ayurveda by Judith H Morrison (Gaia)

Ayurveda – The Gentle Health System by Hans H Rhyner (Sterling)

Ayurveda for Women by Dr Robert E Svoboda (David & Charles)

Perfect Health by Dr Deepak Chopra (Bantam)

Ageless Body, Timeless Mind by Dr Deepak Chopra (Rider)

Ayurveda – A Way of Life by Dr Vinod Verma (Weiser)

The Physiology of Consciousness by Robert Keith Wallace (MIUP)

Body, Mind and Sport by John Douillard (Harmony Books)

The Complete Book of Ayurvedic Home Remedies by Vasant Lad (Piatkus)

Dhanwantari – A Complete Guide to the Ayurvedic Life by Harish Johari (Healing Arts Press)

The Ayurvedic Cookbook by Amadea Morningstar (Lotus Press)

BEAUTY

Absolute Beauty by Pratima Raichur (Bantam)

Beauty Wisdom by Bharti Vyas (Thorsons)

BREATHING

Breathing into Life by Bija Bennett (Hazeldon)

The Breath Book by Stella Weller (Thorsons)

YOGA

Yoga for Stress Relief by Swami Shivapremanda (Gaia)

Yoga Therapy by Stella Weller (Thorsons)

The Yoga Book by Stephen Sturgess (Element)

Dynamic Yoga by Godfrey Devereux (Thorsons)

CRYSTALS

The Book of Crystal Healing by Liz Simpson (Gaia)

MEDITATION

The Three Minute Meditator by David Harp with Nina Feldman (Piatkus)

Mindfulness Meditation for Everyday Life by Jon Kabat-Zinn (Piatkus)

Finding the Stillness Within in a Busy World by Sue Vaughan (Daniel)

HYDROTHERAPY

The Complete Book of Water Therapy by Dian Dinchin Buchman (Keats)

NATURE

The Healing Energies of Water by Charlie Ryrie (Gaia)

The Healing Energies of Trees by Patrice Bouchardon (Gaia)

Tree Wisdom by Jacqueline Memory Paterson (Thorsons)

Healing Herbs by Leslie Kenton (Ebury Press)

Plant Spirit Medicine by Eliot Cowan (Swan, Raven and Co)

PRAYER

How Prayer Heals by Walter Weston (Hampton Roads)

Healing Others by Walter Weston (Hampton Roads)

The God Experiment by Russell Stannard (Faber)

RITUALS

Festivals, Family and Food by Diana Carey and Judy Large (Hawthorn Press)

Rituals for Sacred Living by Jane Alexander (Thorsons)

Everyday Rituals and Ceremonies by Lorna St Aubyn (Piatkus)

Altars Made Easy by Peg Streep (Harper SanFrancisco)

Altars by Denise Linn (Rider)

SPACE CLEARING

Spirit of the Home by Jane Alexander (Thorsons)

The Smudge Pack by Jane Alexander (Thorsons)

Space Clearing by Denise Linn (Ebury Press)

VASTU SHASTRA

Handbook of Vastu by B Niranjan Babu (UBSPD)

INSPIRATIONAL READING FOR PANCHAKARMA

Mudras: Yoga In Your Hands by Gertrud Hirschi (Weiser) would be ideal. Practicing these "finger power points" – yoga positions for hands and fingers – would be a nice quiet practice during restful times.

Creating the Work you Love by Rick Jarow (Destiny Books) – perfect if you're not sure if you're in the right work, this book argues for finding your true calling. The exercises are based on the chakras so it has a nice tie-in with Indian philosophy.

EcoYoga by Henryk Skolimowski (Gaia) – a beautiful little book with practical exercises and meditations for living in harmony with the Earth. Calm, wise, and perfect for detoxing retreats.

Handbook for the Soul edited by Richard Carlson and Benjamin Shield (Piatkus). Often when you're detoxing you don't feel up to reading a whole book, so this collection of essays is ideal for dipping in and out of.

USEFUL ADDRESSES

Ayurvedic Company of Great Britain, 50 Penywern Road, London SW5 9SX (020 7370 2255)

Maharishi Ayur-Veda Health Centre, 21 Clouston Street, Glasgow G20 8QR (0141 946 4663)

Ayurvedic Living, PO Box 188, Exeter EX4 5AB. Provides information on all aspects of Ayurveda – lifestyle, self-help groups, practitioners etc. Please send a large SAE.

Ayurvedic Medical Centre, 1079 Garrett Lane, Tooting, London SW17 02N (020 8682 3876)

Ayurvedic Medical Association UK, The Hale Clinic, 7 Park Crescent, London W1N 3HE (020 7631 0156)

European Ayur-Veda, Hoar Cross Hall, Nr Yoxall, Staffordshire DE13 8QS (01283 575671)

Yoga: The British Wheel of Yoga, 1 Hamilton Place, Boston Road, Sleaford, Lincolnshire NG34 7ES (01529 306851)

Pranayama: The LIFE Foundation School of Therapeutics, Maristowe House, Dover Street, Bilston, West Midlands WV14 6AL (01902 409164)

Meditation: For details of transcendental meditation centers in the UK telephone 0990 143733

Retreats: The Retreat Company, The Manor House, Kings Norton, Leicestershire, LE7 9BA (0116 2599211) www.retreat-co.co.uk
Contact for details of various kinds of retreats – including ayurvedic retreats.

Ayurvedic Medical Clinics: Herbal Holiday Resorts (vt) Ltd. 215/22/Nawala Road, Nugegoda, Sri Lanka.
Tel: 00 94 1 811 422
Kappad Beach Resort, Kozhikode, Kerala, India.
Tel: 00 91 496 683 760 www.kappadbeachresort.com
Kapl Ayurgram, Whitefield, Banglore, Kanataka, India.
Tel: 00 91 080 5591
The Taj Malabar, Cochin, Kerala, India.
Tel: 00 91 484 666 811

Organizations: California College of Ayurveda, 117A East Main Street, Grass Valley, CA 95945. www.ayurvedacollege.com

INDEX

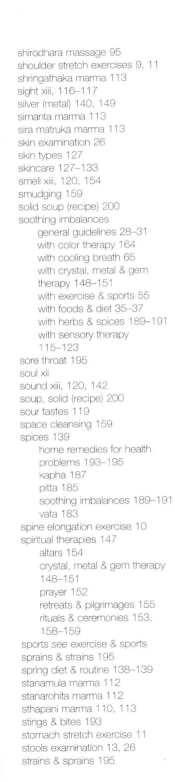

Ville de Montréal

**Feuillet
de circulation**

À rendre le

06.03.375-8 (01-03)